What Others Are Sayin *When You*

A must read for anyone truly interested in furthering their self awareness and wanting to move past fear and resistance to experiencing love in every moment. In so doing, you will be transported to a new way of living with ultimate joy and stop searching for someone outside of yourself to fulfill you!
   ~**Ashley Mann, Alchemical Hypnotherapist,**
Transformational Life Coach, Motivational Speaker and author, recently published in *How to Talk to Your Kids About the Law of Attraction* and *Living the Law of Attraction*

If you want a Soul Mate, you need to become the kind of person you wish to attract. In *You Find Your Soul Mate When You Let Go of Searching*, Gabriella uses stories, examples and exercises to remind the world of this important, and often overlooked, truth.
   ~**Brian Piergrossi**
Life Coach, Spiritual Teacher and author of the book, *The Big Glow: Insight, Inspiration, Peace and Passion*
www.thebigglow.com

A lot of counseling comes down to simply helping a person get out of their own way. Gabriella does a fantastic job of making us aware of how we subconsciously create barriers from that Perfect relationship, how we can break though our obstacles, and how we can achieve what we have always wished for.
   ~**Jason Shoup, Hypnotherapist**

The vital and timely message in Gabriella's transmission is of the highest vibration, and anyone who is seriously seeking their Soul Mate should incorporate the wisdom, grace, and elegance of the techniques developed in this literary work of art. Gabriella's insights touch on the core issues and challenges facing beloveds in today's fast paced high pressure world, and offers practical and inspired advice sure to give you that quantum leap forward you've been looking for. You will enjoy each and every word of this must have volume of divine feminine understanding, and will quickly find yourself rising in love.

~DreamingBear Baraka Kanaan
Spoken Word Artist, Peace Advocate, author of 8 books, including *Wild Love ~Kissed into Consciousness~*

Gabriella gives a unique and warm perspective to the process of awakening your unconscious mind into the infinite consciousness and the being of I am.

~Ford, author of *Becoming God* **and Multi-Platinum Selling Recording Artist**

In *You Find Your Soul Mate When You Let Go of Searching*, you'll learn that there are infinite chances to find your Soul Mate along your lifetime and that every relationship you've ever had, even the disappointing ones, have steered you in the right direction, to understand yourself and experience true love. So, go ahead and dream big! Imagine the most amazing, grandest and most rewarding relationship you could ever have and use the principles in this book to make that your reality.

~ Mike Angulo, Life Coach and Author of the *Eflexx Method for Self-Mastery*
www.eflexx.com

You Find Your Soul Mate When You Let Go of Searching

♥

Gabriella Hartwell

Copyright © 2008 by Gabriella Hartwell

Cover Design by Jennifer Niziankowicz
www.shopsweetums.com

All rights reserved. No part of this book may be reproduced or transmitted in any form or by any means without permission by the author.

ISBN 978-0-6152-3853-1

Your task is not to seek for love, but merely to seek and find all the barriers within yourself that you have built against it.
~Rumi

CONTENTS

Introduction: Perfection is Always Right Now....16

Part One: Truth and Connection
The Search……………………………………….. 22

Truth of Soul Mates…………………………….26

Becoming Aware of Your Self………………………...32

Becoming Aware of Your Soul Mate……………….49

Part Two: Letting Go
Ego: Let Go of the Rope………………………..58

Fear: The Wall which Blocks Manifestation……….67

Releasing the Past……………………………….91

Releasing the Future……………………………97

Releasing Pain……………………………………101

The Power of Gratitude……………………………107

Part Three: Steps to Take to Attract Your Soul Mate
Believe It, Feel It, Know It, Act on It………………...120

Live in the Moment……………………………….124

Notice the Signs and Follow Them………………......128

Part Four: What a Soul Mate Relationship Will Feel Like
Communication with Understanding and Love....134

There Will Be No Doubt....................................136

Height Will Not Be a Factor............................137

The Mirror of Each Other...............................138

Unconditional Love...140

Marriage: A New Beginning............................144

Part Five: What a Soul Mate Relationship Will Look Like
Energies Will Be Similar..................................150

The Presence of Love: Inviting to Others...............151

You Choose Your Own Destiny.........................153

Prayers...157

About the Author...168

Note

To avoid using the masculine gender exclusively when referring to both male and female readers, masculine and feminine pronouns have been randomly used throughout the book.

Acknowledgements

Life is a beautiful journey. First, I want to thank myself for believing in the power of love as well as the power *of* believing. We are all connected and we are all one. Therefore, I am in the utmost gratitude for all who have believed with me and those who have not. It is in our challenges that we grow. It is through our challenges that we are able to profoundly connect with unconditional love. We grow by letting go.

Everyone that has joined their energies into this project in a collaboration to spread the light to the world, I thank you. This is only the beginning!

To all that have been a part of my life and all that will be a part of my life, I thank you for adding to who I am. We are co-creators on the journey of experiencing heaven on earth together.

To my mother: You have become my best friend. Through your support and your unwavering faith in my dreams, you have helped them to come true. You are part of the light that shines through me. Thank you for your love.

To my family: You have all inspired me in your own unique ways. Thank you for choosing to join me through the experiences of life.

Finally, but certainly not least, to my Soul Mate. Your essence strengthens my own, your beauty intensifies my own, your light brightens my own. I know that you are on your way to me, and *very* soon, I will be able to physically embrace you. In your eyes, I am.

To My Readers

My intention with the creation of this book is that you will connect to the beautiful light of love within you. By connecting with this love, you are open to experiencing love with another. You cannot share what you do not have.

You may have the desire to skip over the exercises in this book. If you are serious about connecting with your Soul Mate and you truly want to experience that love, you will give yourself the time to do all of these exercises. It is in doing these that you will become more aware of yourself, which is essential for drawing your Soul Mate to you.

My hope is that you are always lovingly co-creative with others in your relationships. May you be in a state of gratitude for all that you have in your life, all that you have experienced, and all that you are. You are a beacon of light. Let your light shine. When you do, the other half of that light will recognize you.

All my love,
Gabriella

Gratitude is when memory is stored in the heart and not in the mind.
~Lionel Hampton

The Essence of Love

"Love is what makes the world go round," the wise ones say.
Love inspires, it teases, it embraces, we want it to stay. Love thrives, and causes growth, allows for transformation.
Love draws us to the divine, and reminds us of our spiritual connection.
Love anticipates all that is beautiful, requires its essence.
Love enfolds us within its wings, makes known its presence.
There is no escaping this truth: love is what makes us who we are.
Love is what we long for, we will not stop until we hold it within our hearts.
Love is natural, love is created without our awareness, it is what we know.
Love is profound, love allows us to be happy with ourselves, comforted by the afterglow of its reality.

Love is within you, love is within me, love is connecting us, it has always been our history.
Love is our future, it is our present, it is all that we are made of, it will guide us into eternity.
Love is our past, it is existing within each moment, it is what beats within our breast, leading us to ecstasy.
Love will never cease its persistence, it is our calling, it is our peace, pushing us into destiny.
Listen when you hear its voice, it may be soft, it may be a whisper, but it is strong, it will be clear.
Love will remain when you give up, it will remind you that you cannot be anything other than itself.
Love is within you, love is within me, love is connecting us, it has always been our history.
Listen when you hear its voice, it may be quiet, it may be gentle, but it is there, it is in front of you.
Love reminds you always, that it has never forsaken you, it is comfort, it is true.

You may be blind, you may not believe it, though love will never disappear.

Listen to the wisdom that lives within silence, it is love's home, it is where we release fear.
Love is within you, love is within me, love is connecting us, it has always been our history.

Introduction:
Perfection is Always Right Now

I want you to be clear as to what I mean when I use the term "Soul Mate" in this book. Soul Mate is used in our world very often. It's a common term. When people hear the word Soul Mate, automatically a reference goes to a relationship that you have with another soul that is perfect. It is viewed like there is no disruption at all. There is complete harmony all the time. This is true (especially if there was perceived difficulties) because everything that you are experiencing at the time you are experiencing it, is perfect. It's perfect for your growth, in relationship with yourself as well as with other people. It's perfect because it helps you to see parts of yourself that you like and that you may want to change. It also helps you to see the other person you are choosing to be in a relationship with, the things that you want and the things that you don't want.

I believe that you do have more than one Soul Mate within your lifetime. Every person has served a purpose in your life, has helped your soul to grow and you have helped that person's soul to grow, even if the relationship was hard and challenging, *especially* if it was difficult. At the time that you chose to be in a relationship with somebody, that person was your Soul Mate. Soul Mate in this sense does not mean that that relationship will last forever in this lifetime but you have been an elemental part of each other's growth.

Every relationship that you have had, every romantic relationship that you have had has prepared you to receive the ultimate divine connection in a relationship with someone. The Soul Mate that I refer to in the following sections is the Soul Mate that you are ready for once you have gone through other Soul Mate relationships. This connection will happen when your soul has evolved to the point of being ready to merge your whole essence with another, where the focus is truly on love and respect; giving to each other, giving to the world, being a partnership together in service to the world and service to each other. This is the type of Soul Mate love I am referring to.

In this sense, everything will be perfect. All of who you are will match this other person perfectly. You will feel as if this person is the other half of who you are. When you speak to each other, you won't feel a need to explain each other. You will understand where you are both coming from. You will always treat each other with respect and love. There will be no abuse. If the ego does come through at any point in time throughout your relationship, which it may, you will then bring it to the other person's attention and he will realize it. It will be released. The way that you communicate with each other will be completely different from any relationship that you have had in the past.

Everything will be more evolved. That Soul Mate you will find when you let go of searching.

You will want to let go of the search when you are ready, when you are ready to meet this Soul Mate. When you are ready to embrace this soul, you will no longer *want* to search. You will want to be happy with yourself, be happy doing what it is you enjoy and you will emit that type of energy that you want to attract. Therefore, that soul will have to come to you because she will be attracted to you. She will be attracted to the energy that you are putting out into the universe.

This may take some time and you will have to learn patience. It may take some time because that soul also needs to be ready, needs to be ready to embrace you. In order for him to do that, in order for him to recognize you, he needs to go through other relationships. He needs to go through other experiences within his life so that those experiences prepare him for the relationship with you. One of you, either him or you, may still need some experience before you can be together. At that time, you may feel a little bit of anxiety. You want to be there right now. At those moments, patience will sustain you.

It's very important to be patient. This is why it is important to be comfortable with yourself, to have fun on your own. Then, you will be able to live in a very patient state, a calm patient state knowing that she is on her way to you, that your Soul Mate is on her way to you. That knowing, that complete confirmation in your soul only draws your Soul Mate to you. There is power in believing. There is power in letting go of searching.

Part One: Truth and Connection

The Search

When you let go of searching, everything falls into place.
~Gabriella Hartwell
♥

    Our world right now is very focused on searching. We live in a fast forward world. We go to fast food restaurants, drive thrus to get our food as quick as possible. When we have a desire, we want the result to quench our desire as fast as possible. We're searching and searching and searching but we don't want to search for long. We want the search to be quick so that we can satisfy our desires. The same thing goes with finding a Soul Mate or being in the presence of your Soul Mate. We want it quick. When we have the desire, we want to quench it. We want to fulfill it. We go into any type of dating service. We go to a website. We place an ad in the paper. We go to bars. We go anywhere, always searching.

    Let's talk about searching. Searching doesn't allow you to be in the present moment. Searching is always for the future. You are looking to be with someone for the future. You are not focusing on where you are right now in your life. You are not allowing yourself to be content with yourself by yourself. Instead you are looking outside of yourself to find somebody to be in your company so that you can be happy. But happiness comes from within you. You find happiness when you are doing things you enjoy, when you are just *being* and having fun. That's being in the moment. When you are being in the moment and having fun with yourself, doing whatever you are doing by yourself you are attracting the person that you want to attract. You are cultivating the energy that will draw the other half of you *to* you.

When you are searching and you are putting out the energy in the universe that you are searching, you say, *I am not happy with who I am. I am not happy by myself. I am not happy with my life. Therefore I'm looking outside of myself for somebody so that my life can be happy, so that I can be happy.* You will only attract at that time somebody else who is not happy, somebody else who is not happy with himself and his own company, who is also searching.

When you are on a search, you are not focused on what is happening right now in your present moment. You are looking for the next thing and the next thing and the next thing and the next thing. There will always be a continuous search. But when you are just being, and you are having fun by merely existing, then you cultivate other people to you that also are *being* and having fun in life. It is then when you can truly choose somebody who comes to you. You are not looking outside yourself to be happy. You know that you are happy with who you are. That person who is also happy with who she is then comes to you. You both choose to be together to have fun and enjoy life together. The search takes away from that. It is essential to be in the present moment for the manifestation of your Soul Mate within your life. It is in *not* searching that this person will come to you. You will then finally be in the presence of your Soul Mate.

♥

The law of attraction states that you have to think about what it is that you want, you have to think about the person that you want to attract and that person will come to you. This is true however there is an additional part of this. You have to think it, yes, but you also have to feel it. You have to feel the excitement and the desire behind meeting this person. You also have to notice the signs that the universe gives you of the steps to take to manifesting your Soul Mate to you. There *will* be action to take. You are not meant to just sit in your home and just put the thought out there of that person, believe that person is coming to you and do nothing about it.

Once you put that intention out into the universe, the universe will then correspond to what that intention is. It will send people to you. It will send situations to you, opportunities to you. Then you need to recognize those people, those situations, those opportunities that come to you and take the step that you are guided to take. Perhaps it is going to a party that someone invites you to, if that is your feeling behind it, that you should do that. You may be guided to go somewhere else or do something like join a certain club, something that you feel inspired to do. There will be action but the exciting thing here is that the action will be fun. It will be exciting. However, you may have to confront fear. If you like to be at home and you would rather do things at home instead of going to parties, if interacting with a bunch of people is not something that you usually do, you may have to confront the fear of those activities. Let go of the worry about what someone may think, say or how you are going to act, whatever it is that may be stopping you, that may be coinciding with fear in you. You need to let those things go.

Believe that everything is going to turn out fine and everything *will* turn out fine. By taking these steps, being this aware, there is no way your Soul Mate will not be drawn to you. You have all the support of the universe. You have all the support within you.

Truth of Soul Mates

What we call luck is the inner man externalized. We make things happen to us.
~Robertson Davies

♥

What do you know about Soul Mates? Have you heard that it requires just luck to find your Soul Mate and that not many people have that experience in their lifetime? I am here to tell you to discard all of those ideas about luck. Luck has nothing to do with being with the other half of you. Luck is expressing that there is an element of lack. Luck is for people who believe that they have no control over life. Luck is for people that believe things that happen to them just happen for they get whatever life throws at them. The truth is that you *do* have control over your life and your destiny. You are not lucky or unlucky when things happen to you. You are creating everything that you experience and the people that are in your life. If you don't like your experiences, you can change them. If you don't like the company you keep, you can change them.

When you accept the belief that it is rare to encounter your Soul Mate in the physical form and that only a few people ever have this experience on earth, you are setting yourself up to not ever experience this type of blissful love. The truth is that you are not lacking your Soul Mate in your life – your Soul Mate is within you. You just have to connect with yourself. When you do that, you can connect with your Soul Mate and draw him to you in the physical.

♥♥♥♥

You do not have to "find" this person but rather connect with her. To do this, you need to first connect with yourself and realize who you are, what you desire. You need to enjoy your own company and know that your happiness comes from within you. When you know yourself and who you desire, put intention into the universe. The universe will respond. The universe will give you signs. Your job is to notice the signs and follow the steps on your path towards your Soul Mate. You will be brought together at the perfect time for the both of you.

Along the journey to your Soul Mate, there are going to be times when you get anxious, when you want to be with him right now. You may have heard about divine timing. What divine timing means is that everything is happening in your life and in your Soul Mate's life right at this moment to lead you to each other. You have to go through a process so that you can truly let him in your life without anything in the past or future to close you off. He has to go through a process so that he can truly let you into his life.

This is one reason why it is a good thing to practice being with yourself to establish comfort being by yourself and happiness doing things on your own. Overall, that emotion will sustain you in the times when you get anxious, when you want to be with her right now. Feel those emotions. Allow yourself to feel those emotions. They will only strengthen the amount of joy and gratitude you feel when you are finally, physically in the arms of your Soul Mate. It will strengthen that bond.

When you get those feelings, do something creative. Write something, participate in sports, go and do something that gets the energy out, even exercising. Write a letter to that person. Tell him how you feel. Get the energy out but allow yourself to feel those emotions. It is ok to feel those emotions. Sometimes, we have those anxious moments and that does not necessarily mean that we are lonely in the sense that we can't be on our own and be happy. Sometimes there are lonely moments that come up. The difference between not being able to be on your own and be happy versus being on your own but having an anxious, lonely moment is that when you are not comfortable with your own company, you are always looking outside yourself for happiness. You don't feel like you can be doing your own thing, hanging out with your friends, doing pretty much *anything* without a significant other. You also see yourself looking at couples with resentment.

When you are happy and comfortable in your own company and are living in the moment, you are then able to see couples expressing love and be happy for them. You know that your time is coming soon but there may be a time when you are feeling lonely and you just want to feel someone's arms around you, particularly your Soul Mate. That is ok. That is not something that remains with you. You feel it, it happens, recognize it and then let it go. You then get back to who you, back to being happy. That is the difference.

You can't make a mistake in your life. Everything you experience you are to learn from. It makes you who you are, and the same thing for your Soul Mate. He needs to go through things that he is going through too so that you can be together in the way that you envision. It will happen. It is happening right now as you confirm it to yourself. It *is* happening. Don't get discouraged in those moments when you feel lonely. It is a natural human feeling and it will pass. It will help you to appreciate that person so much more when the time comes for you to be together.

Your future is going to turn out the way that you want as long as you approach it with the right attitude of positive belief, you can make anything happen! The first step is determining what it is you want, and then let the universe guide you to manifesting it within your life. The first step to bringing your Soul Mate to you in the physical is to get to know who you are. The second step is to determine who it is you want and then release it into the universe. The universe will then deliver this person to you and you will be able to recognize her when she is standing before you. Be silent enough to notice the signs that are given to you.

Signs can be confusing. I get asked many times how to notice the signs that the universe is sending. The first step is to be aware that signs are around you. There are many signs around us, every single day. If we are not aware of this, we won't be able to notice them. Be aware that there are signs all around you, every day, all the time, everywhere you are. The second step is to notice them. Allow yourself to look around whenever you go somewhere. Allow yourself to recognize where you are, what happens throughout your day. If there are coincidences, those are signs. The word coincidence is another way of saying signs. It's something that happens that seems random but yet when you notice it, it seems not random. It is something that happened that has meaning for you because of how you feel, when you notice that it correlates with something in your life. That makes it a coincidence. That makes it a sign.

After you notice it, and you notice the relevance of it in your life, the next step is to recognize how you feel when you realize the connection. How do you feel? Does it confirm something you believe? Does it confirm some action that you were feeling you should take? Perhaps it could be the opposite in confirming something you were questioning or warning you of going ahead with something you were considering. But it is important to notice the feelings that go along with the sign.

This is another reason why patience is so important. It could happen that you get one sign. You go somewhere or talk to someone and instantly, your Soul Mate is there but there may be more than one sign that leads you to your Soul Mate. This means that you have to have the patience to constantly live in this type of way and be content knowing that it may not be the first sign that brings you to your Soul Mate. You have the trust in knowing that there will be other signs. You just follow. That is your job.

The thing about signs is to notice when the universe sends you them, which is mainly to be aware of your surroundings, the people that come to you, the situations you are in, etc. What you have to be aware of is the feelings behind the signs when you notice them.

The final step is to take action. If this sign has caused you to feel that you need to take a step or go somewhere or talk to someone, then your next step is to follow, to take that action. There is not just going to be one. There is going to be many. There is going to be consistent signs on your path and your journey of life. When you are aware that there are signs, you recognize them, pay attention to how you feel when you recognize them. Then you take the action that you are guided to take. There will then be another sign, and there will be another sign, and there will be another sign. You will have consistent guidance on your path and your journey of life, on your path and your journey to your Soul Mate.

Becoming Aware of Your Self

The more you are the love you want to attract, the easier it will be for that love to recognize you.
~Gabriella Hartwell
♥

If you have been struggling with love, it is time to let the struggle go. If you have been drowning in a sea of negativity and doubt in your relationships, it is time to let the negative and the doubts go. If you believe that you are not good enough, beautiful enough, experienced enough to have the love you desire, it is time to let go of those beliefs. It has always been the time to let go.

The truth is: there is no struggle in love. There is no negativity and doubt in love. You are more than good enough, beautiful enough and experienced enough in love to be able to let yourself have and enjoy the love you are craving. You can have this love whether you are single or are currently in a romantic relationship.

How can you do that? The first step is getting to know what makes you tick, what you are passionate about, what echoes so profoundly within your soul, who you are. Have you ever thought about what your true feelings are on life, how you approach life? For example, do you wake up and feel that the day is going to be great, that you have many opportunities to experience happiness or do you approach a new day as if it is exhausting, that you can't wait until it's over so that you can end it? Do you have a smile on your face throughout the day or does it seem like a chore to have a positive attitude? Do you feel as though you are helped, loved, and appreciated throughout your day or do you feel as though no one cares and you are in a universe all by yourself? It is extremely important to understand and connect with the truth of who you are and how you approach life.

Life Exercise

Write a list of the ways in which you view life, the ways in which you approach each new day, and the feelings that come up when you think about life.

If you noticed that you have some negative views on life, let's turn that around. How can you change the negative views to positive ones? Affirmations are a reversal of a negative feeling or thought that you repeatedly tell yourself. It is something that subconsciously you want to believe and by repeating the affirmation, you tend to start feeling it, and therefore can change the way you think about something. Example: Life does not offer me any opportunity to be happy = life offers me many opportunities to be happy. Example: I wake up feeling tired = I wake up refreshed and ready to embrace the day. So, look again at the list above and make your own affirmation list below, turning the negative statements into positive ones, affirmations. If you noticed that your list has all positive statements, then put them down under the affirmations. This way you are confirming them to yourself.

Affirmations

Your approach on life will need to be similar to your Soul Mate so that you can be compatible. For example, if you are positive and an optimistic person, you see anything that happens in life in a positive light and the person you are with sees life as negative and always focuses on the negative aspect within an experience, your outlooks are not compatible. This may cause resentment towards each other and if one of you will not change the way you view life, it may not work. The way that you view life needs to be similar. You need to be operating on the same frequency.

There is also such a thing as a vacation style. For example, I once dated a gentleman who always had to be moving and always had to be doing something. When we would go camping, he would always have to be doing something. He couldn't just sit and relax and enjoy relaxing. He had to be doing some type of activity: playing Frisbee, taking a walk on the beach. He could not sit down and relax on the beach, always had to be in movement.

If you do not have the same vacation style, how you approach relaxation, how you approach the times when you allow yourself to get away from all responsibilities, if those are different, your energies may not be compatible. One way that you could work this out would be if you both compromise. He will relax like you want to relax and vice versa. You will do an activity with him as well. But when you come in contact with your Soul Mate, the way that you approach relaxation will be the same. You will be very compatible.

Write down what vacation means to you, how you like to relax.

My Vacation Style

You may have thought of what you wanted your Soul Mate to do for a job. I don't believe that it is important to have the specific job title in mind and that's only what you accept. Your careers, the way you handle work, needs to be compatible with each other. For example, if you have a job that involves creating: writing movie scripts, writing songs, writing a book, acting, any type of creative job, you need to know how you approach that work.

If you have a creative job, and you know that you need to have time away from your partner at times to be able to create, then your partner is going to need to understand that. If that person also has a job where she needs to create, then she will understand the need to be away at times. You will allow each other the space to create but then come together, perhaps create together or just *be* together. The style in which you work is an important thing. It is essential to understand that about yourself in order to know if it is compatible with someone else that you choose to be with. You won't know if it's compatible if you do not take the time to realize how you work and how you approach work.

Write down how you approach work: do you need time away? Do you work more than 8 hours in a day? What would need to be compatible with someone else in how they approach work or how they understand you in regards to your work?

My Work Approach

Have you thought about your long term goals in life and what is truly important to you? What do you feel is so much a part of who you are? How you approach life should complement the person you want to attract and vice versa. However, your goals need to also match in order for you to live together happily. When these goals are in sync, it supports your spiritual growth while allowing each other to fulfill your dreams and live your life purpose. Love never restricts another from being happy. Love wants to see the other person happy, even if the both of you need to be physically apart at times to fulfill your life mission.

Below, write a list of what is important to you in relation to your future goals: in your career, personal life, etc. Ex. Helping others within my work.

Future Goals Exercise

Be aware that if helping others is important to you, your Soul Mate will not feel that people should help themselves. The energy vibration between the both of you will be operating on the same frequency. You can see that this example does not show two people who would be compatible together because this core value is within them, and it differs from the other. The energies need to match to offer an equal balance so that the goals are in sync. Your Soul Mate's future goals *will* match yours perfectly. Your future goals may even coincide so well that you may take on a mission together, intensifying your growth together profoundly.

Our Soul Mate is someone who shares our deepest longings, our sense of direction. When we're two balloons, and together our direction is up, chances are we've found the right person.
~Richard Bach
♥

Have you ever seen a couple that just seem to complement each other in every way? When one of them is down, the other lifts that person up and vice versa. It's like a seesaw. It's an equal balance of give and take. Have you seen how they laugh together? Have you seen how it seems like they are almost never unhappy? These people may end up doing something together like taking on a mission in the world or their jobs/careers tend to coincide with the other. This is what I am referring to when I talk about your energies matching each other. Your goals will coincide. You may have careers that are different from each other but there is an underlying similarity. For example like I mentioned, you may both have helping professions in some light. If you think about it, there are a lot of jobs and a lot of careers that are helping professions but if you took one or the other, technically they are not the same. If you both feel that helping people is important, that is something that unites you. Your energies are balancing on the same frequency. There is an equal give and take. There is an understanding that doesn't need any words because it is what you both truly feel deep inside your selves. That is the type of energy match I am referring to with your Soul Mate. This is what you will experience.

Have you experienced relationships in the past where there were so many differences, that when you combined both your energies, there was not a match? At the time, it was probably frustrating but it showed you what you do *not* want. That was not the person for you in the long run. Those experiences have given you that lesson and that knowing. There will be no doubt when you meet this other person who is your Soul Mate. It will be very clear to you. All the stars, so to speak, will line up. Everything will match in a perfect way.

♥

Have you ever thought of how you feel about marriage? If you are thinking about attracting and meeting your Soul Mate, marriage must have come up in some form or another. What are your thoughts and feelings regarding marriage? Do you want to get married or not? How do you view marriage, as something to be dreaded, the end of your freedom or do you see it as a beginning, a chance to combine who you are with someone else? If you have decided that you want to get married, how do you envision your married life to be like? If you have decided not to get married, how do you envision your relationship to be like? Write a list of your thoughts about marriage.

Marriage Exercise

Now, take a look at the list you just wrote and repeat all of the statements aloud to yourself. Notice how you feel after each one. Are there any that don't make you feel good? If so, write an affirmation list to change the energy around. If you feel good about all of the statements you wrote, then confirm them by writing them in the affirmation list.

Affirmations

Marriage Visualization Exercise

Now would be a good time to do a visualization exercise regarding your ideas about marriage and the relationship you see yourself in. Visualization takes something you feel and think and transforms it into a movie scene. You have some feelings and thoughts on the relationship you are moving towards and now it is time to take them into a more tangible form. Through this visualization, you will be able to truly confirm to yourself whether what you are feeling and thinking about marriage resonates deep within the core of who you are. To do this exercise, you will need to create a sacred, safe space where you can relax and tune into you. Put on some soft music with no words or keep silence if you are comfortable with that. Allow yourself to get physically comfortable, whether it be in a sitting position or lying down. Close your eyes, and envision yourself at your wedding as you stand beside your partner. Notice how you feel and how the energy is all around you. Notice how he reacts towards you and how everyone else is acting. Are they having fun? Is it a sunny day? Where are you?

Now, let's go a little further. Imagine yourself with this partner three months into your marriage. Where are you living? What are you doing? How are you interacting with each other? Are you laughing and feeling good? Allow yourself to envision further into the future with this person. Are you still laughing and feeling good? Allow yourself to feel those emotions and then slowly open your eyes. Notice if the feelings you experienced throughout the visualization are accurate with what you wrote in the list above or if they are different. Write a list of how you saw your marriage and what you felt while seeing it. Do you still feel the same? If so, reinforce those feelings by writing them below.

Affirmations

It is natural to think of children when marriage is brought up, so let yourself think of how you truly feel about having children. Do you want children? How do you feel when you think about having children? Write a list of your feelings about having children.

My Views on Having Children

Take a look at your list and see if there are any negative statements regarding having children, are there any fears? Take those negative statements and make them positive.

Affirmations

Have you thought about what you feel about raising your children? Do you want them to attend school or be home schooled? What are your thoughts about punishment or do you not believe in punishment? What is important to you that you want to pass on to your children? Write a list of those important things you feel about raising children.

My Views on Raising Children

What are your views on religion and/or spirituality? What are your thoughts on God? What moral values do you strongly believe in? Is it important to you to attend a church/service every week? This may require more than one list – let yourself write as much as you need to regarding all of these questions.

My Moral Values/Views on God and Spirituality

Now that we have looked at some core values that you believe in and feel strongly about, it is now time to focus on the characteristics that make you who you are. These are the traits that you will be bringing to a relationship. We will be going into detail not only of your personality traits, but also the physical traits that make you feel beautiful. The truth is that you are beautiful just the way you are, and your Soul Mate loves you for exactly the way you are. When you connect with this truth, your light shines so brightly and you cannot help but attract the person you desire.

Write a list of the personality traits that you bring to a relationship. There are no limitations here – get a separate piece of paper if you need to. Your only goal in writing this list is to be true to yourself and to what you feel.

Personality Traits Exercise

After looking at the list above, did you notice anything that you wrote which is not a positive trait? If so, take that trait and make it positive. If you notice that the traits you wrote above are positive, confirm them to yourself by writing them again in the list below.

My Positive Traits Exercise

Your friends and your family are a significant part of your support circle, and they can see your positive traits in a different light. You may notice how sometimes your ego comes into play when you are attempting to focus on the positive aspects of who you are, and it is that voice that we will work on later, how to recognize it and let it go. You may be very excited now with these exercises for it is fun getting to know yourself, and spending time in your own company. It is the same amount of fun that others experience when they are around you. How about asking your closest friends and family members what they think are your positive traits? Try asking them to pick one or two positive traits that they notice about you. Write the list below.

My Positive Traits Through the Eyes of Family/Friends

Now, take a look at this list and compare it to the one that you wrote. Are there similar traits or other ones? If there are ones that you didn't include in your list, add them to that list.

♥♥♥♥

In addition to your positive traits, let yourself focus on your physical traits that are unique to you and that make you who you are. You are a being of light and there is beauty within you as well as around you. Your job is to notice that beauty and let it shine. Write down all the physical traits that you find beautiful about you. Perhaps you have naturally curly hair, gentle hands, etc. Have fun with this.

My Physical Traits

Take a look at this list and focus on each trait. Take a walk over to the mirror and look at the beauty that is emanating from your form. Look at all the specific traits that you find beautiful, bask in the energy that is being released from these parts of you. Allow yourself to look at all of who you are. There may be more traits that you notice as you look more thoroughly at yourself in the mirror. Please add these to your list. How do you feel? Close your eyes and take a deep breath. Let yourself feel the energy of being within your own body, the vessel that your soul is dwelling within.

Open your eyes, look at yourself again in the mirror. Say these affirmations below, one at a time, aloud to yourself. Let yourself feel any emotions that come up as you feel the words that you speak.

Affirmations

1. I am light
2. I am beautiful
3. I am unique in my own way
4. I have the ability to heal myself
5. I love myself unconditionally
6. I am worthy to receive love
7. I am able to give love
8. I am alive
9. The essence of who I am is love

Becoming Aware of Your Soul Mate

Lovers don't finally meet somewhere, they're in each other all along.
~Rumi

What have you heard about Soul Mates? This is the time to let go of anything you may have thought you knew about Soul Mates and begin a new idea. It has always been the time to let go. The truth is that you are never separated from your Soul Mate. You have never been away from that other half of your soul. By truly connecting with who you are, all that you believe, all that you are excited about, you are sending out a natural vibration of energy into the universe directly to the other side of who you are, your Soul Mate. The only way that you will come in contact with this person is by connecting to the inner truth and beauty within you.

Since you have done that in the previous chapter, the opportunity is now in front of you to invite your knowledge, your remembrance of this other side of you into your awareness. You are going to do that in a similar way that you approached your knowledge of who you are, by exercises and visualizations.

Remember how you felt when you were visualizing being in the presence of this soul partner. Close your eyes, take a deep breath and feel that energy again. Place yourself back into the image of connecting with that soul, feel the emotions. You are now in the place to connect with the essence that is the other half of you.

Before you start these exercises, it is important to discard any ideas you may have accepted from society or other people on who you should marry or be with. These lists need to resonate within your soul as truth for *you*. The first list is going to focus on the traits that you do not want in a partner. Be completely honest with yourself.

Personality Traits That my Soul Mate Does Not Have

Take a look at that list and notice how you feel when you focus on those traits. When you are envisioning what you want in your life, never keep the focus on the negative. However, the negative and what you don't want can be essential for realizing what it is that you *don't* want so that you can put your energy on what you *want* and attract that to you. Take the list you wrote above and change the negative traits you don't want into positive traits that you do want in a life partner. For example, lying = trustworthy.

Personality Traits that My Soul Mate Possesses

Remember when you wrote the physical traits that you found beautiful with yourself? Here is your chance to make that same list for your Soul Mate. What physical traits will this person have? You can be as specific as you want here, as long as you connect within yourself to that other soul. What does this person look like? For example, brown hair or kind eyes.

Physical Traits of My Soul Mate

At this point, you may be feeling a connection to this person. After all, you can tune into your Soul Mate's energy at any time for you are both a part of each other. Allow yourself to connect more to the energy, and think about the family that you will be joining into. How do you see this family? Is your Soul Mate an only child or are there other siblings? Are the parents divorced, remarried or have the parents been together since this person was born? Write a statement on how you envision this family to be like. This statement can be as long and detailed as you feel.

Statement on My Soul Mate's Family

Have you thought about how this person interacts with friends and family? How does your Soul Mate treat others? Take a moment to relax. Close your eyes, take a deep breath and let yourself travel to where your Soul Mate is in the midst of other people. These other people could be friends, family or coworkers. Your role is to just observe the way that this soul is expressing himself with others. Then, write a statement as detailed as you feel about what you witnessed.

How My Soul Mate Treats Others

What do you feel about finances? How do you envision this person's finances to be like? What is important to you in this area? How do you want him to approach money? Does he need to have a substantial amount of money or does that not matter to you? Truly connect within yourself as to what you feel is important ~ let go of any ideas that you may have accepted from society or others. This statement needs to connect to the truth of what *you* feel.

The Financial Reality of My Soul Mate

This next exercise may cause you to pause for a moment and think as it is an essential part of this whole process. Many people want to be in the presence of that perfect person, their Soul Mate, the one that will complement who they are. Rightly so, there is an inherent craving within to reconnect with that other half of our soul. Before you can come in contact with this person, you need to be clear as to why it is you want this soul's presence in your life. Think about this honestly and write down your truth.

Determine why you truly want to connect with this person. What is your objective? What is your mission, your purpose? If you want someone for sex, you don't need a Soul Mate for that. If you want someone to help you with the housework, you don't need a Soul Mate for that. If you want someone because you are lonely, you don't need a Soul Mate for that. Be very specific with yourself as to the why behind this desire. Write down why it is that you want to come together with your soul partner.

The Reason Behind the Desire of Connecting with My Soul Mate

After you write this statement, you may feel a complete clarification within your soul, an excitement that urges you onward to fulfill the mission of being with this partner. You are now ready to take the next step.

You are going to create an affirmation which includes some of the lists you have made. Look again at the list of personality traits/qualities that you bring to a relationship and also the traits that your Soul Mate possesses. In addition, confirm to yourself the reason why you want to come together with this person.

I, <u>Your Name Goes Here</u>, bring these qualities to a relationship:

I am looking for someone that brings these qualities into the relationship:

We are going to come together for the purpose of
_____.

I will accept ONLY this person as a romantic partner OR someone better.

Surrender, by definition, means letting go of attachment to results.
~Marianne Williamson, <u>A Return to Love</u>.

    The next important step is that you need to put this affirmation and your lists aside, and not look at them again. It has always been the time to let go. By thinking about them and writing them down, you have now put the energy out into the universe. If you were to constantly think about them or compare people you meet to them, you would be placing energy into the possibility that you may not receive what you desire. This is the point where you need to trust. You need to trust that the universe will make things happen so that you come into the presence of this life partner, and that you do not need to focus on these specifics for that to occur. Do not worry about how it will happen for that takes away from energy you need to be putting into yourself, into getting ready for your encounter. It is important for you to make these lists so that you will recognize this particular soul when you are standing before him. Have faith that he is already on his way to you.

Part Two: Letting Go

Ego: Tug of War Can't Continue if You Let Go of the Rope

The ego is not master in its own house.
~Sigmund Freud
♥

Before you can welcome this person into your life, there are some things you need to let go of. It has always been the time to let go. Your ego needs to be silenced. It may never completely leave you, however your job is to recognize its voice and put it into the proper perspective. The ego will attempt to sway you from your goal, try to make you feel that it is impossible, that you don't deserve it, etc. There are simple ways to realize that the ego is at work. If what you hear does not make you feel good, if it places any semblance of doubt into your mind, then that is the ego. You want to be in the place where you hear the voice, but you don't let it change how you feel or stop you from accomplishing your dreams. If you can wrestle right back, the ego will eventually give up because you are not letting it control you.

The ego will not confront you as often as in the beginning of your process of letting it go, however it is important to recognize its voice so that when it does reappear, you will be able to send it back to its proper place. It is not a companion that you want on your journey to living your dreams, for it will only attempt to block your path and your confidence in getting there.

How do you put it in its place? You need to combat the negative words with positive ones. For example:

Ego ~ What are you going to say to people if it doesn't work out?
You ~ It is working out so there is no need to think about this.

Another example:
Ego ~ You have only had unsuccessful relationships, how can you find and keep love?
You ~ I am living in the present moment. I can love, I do love, therefore I can find and keep love.

♥ As a side note, there are no unsuccessful relationships. All relationships served their purpose at the time and there are lessons to learn. There is power in letting go.♥

By doing this, you are shifting your energy to the positive, and keeping your focus there. The universe responds to positive affirmations powerfully and just so, the ego shrinks in the presence of such power. Remember how you felt as a young adolescent standing before a person of authority who was speaking in a strong, commanding tone? You probably felt as if there was no other option for you but to obey. This is the role of the ego when you assert yourself with such conviction. You are in control, and that is where you want to be. Let the ego go. Release its hold on your thoughts, your emotions, your dreams, your path to having the love you desire. You have everything you need to move forward. If you believe and don't let anything come in the way of that belief, you will get to where you want to be.

Think about your life. Are there any instances where you can recall that the ego attempts to control you and not make you feel good? What areas are those? Can you recall the thoughts/beliefs that come up that don't make you feel good? Refer to the example above to write a list of what the ego says to you through your thoughts/emotions and then counteract them with positive powerful statements against it.

Silencing the Ego Exercise

Ego	You

Do you feel powerful after this exercise? You have the power within you to silence the ego when it tries to control you. Always remember that the ego will never make you feel good. There is a variety of emotions behind the words the ego uses; guilt, envy, greed, self-consciousness, fatigue, etc. When you are feeling an emotion that doesn't make you feel good, notice it and try to get at the heart of why you are feeling that way. It may be a belief that is hindering you, that no longer serves you. If you refuse to be controlled, you will not be controlled. If you refuse to feel bad, you will always allow yourself to feel good. Focus on feeling good. Have the confidence to let go. It has always been the time to let go.

"To show you one of life's simple lessons," the alchemist answered. "When you possess great treasures within you, and try to tell others of them, seldom are you believed."
~Paulo Coelho, <u>The Alchemist</u>

♥

Your ego is not only going to come out through your own thoughts and feelings about whatever it is that you are deciding to do or not do. Your ego will also come forth when other people are telling you their thoughts and their feelings about something that you may have decided to do, something that you feel very strongly about. People will challenge you. When people challenge you, your ego gets excited because it has an opportunity to try to control you.

If you tell someone something that you have decided to do, or if you tell someone something about how you feel, that person cannot feel what you feel because that person is *not* you. You can try as hard as you would like to try to explain to them how you feel. They may hear you but they may not understand you or understand where you are coming from. They do not have the feelings behind the words that you say. You know inside yourself of what you feel about what you are choosing to do or what you are choosing to believe. You are the only person that knows your emotions and can feel them.

Your feelings are confirmation that you are on the right path or that you are not on the right path. When you know, no doubt, by your feelings that you are on the right path, another person cannot feel and know without a doubt that you are on the right path. Therefore, it's important to know, you do not need permission from anybody else to do what it is you feel you need to do or to believe whatever it is you feel you need to believe.

When you get excited about something, something that you feel, something that you know, you want to talk about it. It's a natural feeling to want to talk about it. It's a natural part of us to want to share things that we are excited about. But there is a downside to this sharing if you *allow* it to be a downside. Other people are going to tell you their opinions when you express your excitement. Their opinions may be so different from yours. Their opinions may come out in a way that is expressing to you that what you are feeling or what you are believing is crazy, is impossible and there is no way that you can do that.

People will not know your dreams like you do because they can't feel them like you do. You have a choice when you start expressing your excitement to people. You have a choice to take in what they say to you and believe it too. The ego will try to help them have this effect on you. When you hear someone say, "*That's impossible. You can't do that,*" all of a sudden your ego is going to start saying things like, *Gosh, they are right. You can't do this. How could you even think that you could do this?* If it's what you believe, someone may say, "*That's impossible to believe that. It's crazy for you to even think that.*" The ego will then say, *You are crazy and if you go ahead and believe this, and then you take action because of this belief, you are crazy. You are going to fail. There is no way that you are going to be able to do this.* Your job at this point is to silence the ego, counteract it with the positive.

As mentioned before, the positive is very affirmative and it is so much stronger than negative. Light is stronger than darkness in this sense. Counteract it with, *I KNOW I can do this because I FEEL this is what I HAVE to do. I KNOW this is possible because I can SEE it.* You can't show people your visions by expressing your visions in words. People cannot feel and see your visions like you do. There is a knowing inside of you that is for you. It's for you to know that your feelings and your visions are bringing you to where you want to be and to where you need to be. That is for your purpose.

Don't let people change your desire and your belief in your dreams. Your dreams will not be affected unless you *let* them. It is important to have a support system when you are taking the steps in following your dreams and when you are taking the steps towards your Soul Mate. It's important for you to follow the path that you need to be on. When you are following that path, it is very helpful to have a support system of people that are encouraging you and that believe in you as well as your dreams.

Here is where I want to bring in the law of attraction. The law of attraction states that you bring to yourself what it is that you feel. If you are putting out into the universe where you know you want to go, who you want to be with, then the law of attraction is going to bring to you other people who are on their path to manifesting their dreams as well as their Soul Mate relationship. The universe will bring to you people that are thinking and believing as you are. However, you will also have to go through those relationships with people that do not agree with you so that you become stronger in your belief. You can then appreciate the support system that is brought to you more profoundly because you have experienced *not* having that support.

Once again, it is important to realize that those people that challenge you can't change your desire and belief in your dreams. Your dreams will not be affected. The manifestation of your dreams and your Soul Mate will not be affected unless you let them be affected by changing your belief. When you feel something with a knowing sense inside of you, when you even think of not believing in what it is you feel, that will be much more uncomfortable than believing in what you know. People will not know your dreams like you do because they can't feel them like you do. It has always been the time to let go of how other people may perceive you, of how other people may think about your dreams, your beliefs, your feelings, your knowing. It's always been the time to let go of the false need to be accepted by other people. There is power in believing. There is power in knowing. There is power in following the path towards your dreams.

It is only your thinking that your dreams will not happen that creates your dreams from *not* happening. It is only your thinking that you will not come in contact with your Soul Mate that will *not* allow for you to come in contact with your Soul Mate. Once you change your thinking and your feeling about your thoughts, your dreams will manifest and your Soul Mate will be brought to you.

Fear: The Wall which Blocks Manifestation

Death is not the biggest fear we have; our biggest fear is taking the risk to be alive - the risk to be alive and express what we really are.
~Don Miguel Ruiz, <u>The Four Agreements</u>
♥

What is fear? Fear is an extension of the ego. There is a strong connection between fear and the ego. When you hear doubts within you, it is the ego speaking to you. Automatically, you start to feel fear. When you hear, *You won't be able to do that. How could you even think that?* automatically, the fear steps in. You hear things like, *Geez, I don't know why I was thinking this. How am I going to be able to do this? How am I going to be able to accomplish what I want to?* The ego thrives on you being afraid, it thrives on you not having the strength to believe and take the steps in what you believe so that you can manifest what you want to manifest, whatever it is that you are trying to accomplish.

    The ego comes forward with a question or an affirmative negative statement about you, whether it be what you believe, what you are doing or not doing, or just about you in general. It will give you a question like, *How can you think that?* or it will give you an affirmative negative statement like, *You are crazy. That's impossible.* Rather than let fear take over when you hear something like that, your job is to counteract that with a positive question or statement. For example, *How can I not go ahead and do this? It is what I feel so strongly inside.* Anything is possible if you believe in it and feel it.

Fear thwarts your growth and does not allow your dreams to manifest. Fear will stop you from doing what you need to do so that your dreams can fully be manifested within your life, so that your Soul Mate can fully be brought to you. The truth is there is nothing to be afraid of. Anything is possible if you believe it. Your dreams have a way of manifesting. Your dreams have a way of coming true if you believe in them. Let go of fear, counteract your ego with positive statements, positive energy and you are well on your way to manifesting all that you want in your life. There is nothing to be afraid of.

Fear is a negative emotion. There are only two emotions and all other emotions stem from these: love and fear. If you are operating from fear, you are blocked. You are blocked from experiencing love. Fear is the emotion that stops you from doing anything that you enjoy because of something. For example, you want to go to this party but you are afraid that you might not look good, that you might not get the perfect outfit, that people might judge you. You are operating from fear. You don't go to the party perhaps because of fear. It is blocking you from experiencing what you would like to experience. Life is meant to be fun. We are supposed to have fun on this journey. Fun is an important factor. Fear blocks you from having fun.

How does fear block you from having and experiencing the love you desire and that you deserve? You are going to be offered opportunities that are different from what you have experienced in the past. It may be meeting new people, going to places where you can meet new people, even in regards to your career. These people may be different from your experiences in the past as well as these places you are invited to go to. They are new to you. They are a part of the unknown. It is scary, but you can take that fear and you can confront it. It is something that you can go through and by going through it, you become stronger. Then you allow yourself to have fun. You allow yourself to have another experience that life brings you.

If you are afraid, you don't take action. It is necessary to take action to come in contact with your Soul Mate. These actions will be fun. For example, taking care of yourself, going to the gym, getting new clothes, going out and doing things that you enjoy to do even if no one else goes with you, doing those things that you enjoy by yourself, smiling, talking to people that you do not know yet. That can be scary. If you confront fear, and you have it be your ally on your journey of life, then you can get through anything and you can get to your Soul Mate faster.

The essential thing is to be comfortable with yourself so that you can confront fear. Perhaps the fear of what people may think, fear of what people will say, fear of what people will think of what you say or do. You are who you are and you are a beautiful person. You are unique in your own way. Nobody can be you. If anybody puts you down, you don't have to take it personally because it is not against you. Their reaction is because of whatever they are choosing to believe from their experiences within their own life. It is not against you. You are beautiful just the way that you are. You are unique in the ways that you are. You deserve to experience and have the love that you desire. Do not let fear get in the way from experiencing this type of Soul Mate love.

♥

When you see other couples expressing love to each other, do not allow yourself to feel resentment. Resentment comes from fear, fear that you will not be able to experience that love, fear that you will not be lucky as those people are lucky in love. Remember that luck equals lack. You are not lacking anything. The truth is you are experiencing that love *with* yourself and in turn, you will be attracting that love from someone else, who is your Soul Mate. It is just a matter of time before you have that expression of Soul Mate love. You wouldn't want someone else to pass you while you are in that relationship, and be resentful because that would not make you feel good, if you knew they were being resentful. When you are happy, you want to remain happy. You don't want anything to change your energy or anyone to change your energy. You want to stay happy. You would want people to be happy for you and even if you have single friends, you wouldn't want them to play the victim. You wouldn't want them to say things to you like, "*I'll never have that love or that love will never find me,*" when you are expressing your happiness. You would want them to be happy for you, to say things like, "*Congratulations, I am so happy you found your Soul Mate. I know I can have that love too and I will be experiencing that soon.*" It is a different reaction and a different feeling behind those words than when someone is feeling resentment towards people that are happy and in that type of relationship.

The truth of the matter is that it really is only time. It is only a matter of time before you are in that relationship. There is no need to focus on how much time and when it is going to happen because that takes you away from the moment. All you need to do is enjoy your life and be happy. You need to do everything that you can to enjoy your life and be happy. Let fear go or take it along for the ride with you. Recognize it. Fear is an extension of the ego. Recognize it, take it with you, dance with it. You can have fun with this. You can realize how you feel when the emotion or thought of fear comes up. You can say, "*Yes, I recognize this and I'm going to let it go. I am going to **let... it... go**.*" It has always been the time to let go.

Fear is only an illusion. It is not the truth. There is truly nothing to be afraid of. You are beautiful. You are perfect the way that you are. You are living the life you are choosing to live and you can change it if you do not like it. There is no need to be afraid of being alone. Loneliness itself is an illusion. All you need to be happy is realizing that you are already happy with yourself, and allowing yourself to be happy in your own company.

You are happiness. Happiness comes from within you. You do not need anyone for your own happiness. That's a false illusion. Whitney Houston sang in her song, "It's Not Right but It's Ok" a line that is very relevant here: "I'd rather be alone than unhappy." This is a statement of profound truth. Why be in a relationship just to be in a relationship and be unhappy? Think of all the exciting things you could be doing instead and how by doing those things, you could be getting closer and closer to the soul that you are meant to be with. When you are emitting positive energy just by having fun, you are attracting that same type of energy back to you.

When you are physically alone, you are never alone. Get past the idea that when you are *physically* alone with yourself, that you *are* alone. Alone is all a state of mind. The thoughts about being alone need to change if you want to be in a Soul Mate relationship.

What do you feel when you think of not being in a relationship at any given time? Are you ok with being in your own company without another person or do you feel lonely at that time? Where is this loneliness coming from? Joy comes from within and therefore, you create happiness with anything that you do. Loneliness is an illusion.

When you are physically alone, you are never alone. When you are feeling that you are alone in your own presence, if you attract a significant other into your life during that time, the person that you are attracting will also feel that same way. He will feel that he cannot be alone. He will feel that when he is physically alone, he is alone and he will not like that feeling, as you do not like that feeling. Therefore, you will spend so much time with each other because you are afraid of being alone. Even if that relationship is abusive in some form, you will stay together because you are afraid of being alone.

When you come from a place where you are happy in your own presence, you then have the opportunity to make a choice. You can choose to be with this person or you do not because you are not afraid of being alone. If you do end a relationship, you will be physically alone again. The truth is *that is ok*. There's nothing wrong with being physically alone. The only thing that is stopping you from being alone in your own presence and being ok with that is fear; fear of not finding a relationship, fear of not having that love. If you recall the voice of the ego and how it may say that you will never experience this type of love, you can counteract that.

Yes, you WILL experience that type of love. There is NO reason for you not to be ok with being alone right now.

Fear only distracts you from having everything that you want. It doesn't allow you to focus on the life that you want, the person that you want to be and attracting the person that you desire. Fear is an extension of the ego. Fear is a way that the ego tries to control you. All you need to do is change your thoughts on it. Change your thoughts on being alone. Alone is all a state of mind. When you are physically alone, you are never alone.

If you find that you are staying in an abusive relationship because it is familiar, you need to change that belief, that underlying belief that you deserve that kind of treatment. It is familiar to you for it is what you have allowed. You have allowed that person to treat you in an abusive way because somewhere inside you feel you deserve to be treated like that. That is not the truth. You can change that belief. You deserve to be treated with love. You are worthy of love. The truth is, if you believe in yourself and you love yourself, others will as well. If you believe in yourself, others will believe in you as well. If you love yourself, others will love you as well.

The reverse of this is when you don't believe in yourself and you don't love yourself, then others will also treat you like that. There will be a little bit of restriction in a way. You will complain about it. You will not be happy with this type of treatment. Deep down inside, you know that you deserve better than that and it is that deep down inside feeling that you need to connect with. When you connect with that feeling, you will not allow anybody to treat you with disrespect and without love.

The unfamiliar can be scary. To be treated with that intense amount of love and respect can be scary in a way if you have not experienced it before. It is something that you are not familiar with. If you really and truly allow yourself to envision being in that type of relationship, the amount of comfort is so strong, the amount of love is SO strong. Ultimately, that is what you desire. That is what your soul craves for. Do not stay in an abusive relationship. You don't deserve that. If you believe in yourself, others will as well. If you love yourself, others will as well.

Why is it better to be alone than unhappy? Write a statement on why you feel that it is better to be alone than unhappy in a relationship.

Single versus Unhappy in a Relationship

Can you recall a situation where you were unhappy in a relationship? Write that down. Why were you unhappy? Why were you unhappy in this relationship?

The Reason Behind an Unhappy Relationship

Take a look at this reason. Recall the situation. Recall this relationship to your memory. How would it have been different if you were alone and not with this person? How would your experience of life have been different at that time?

I'm going to relay an experience that I have had in a previous relationship. I was with someone where it would be one sided. He would suggest and make the plans of what we would do. When we would go out and do these activities that he suggested, he would be fine, he would be happy and he approached whatever we did in a positive way. We were doing what he wanted to do. Whenever I suggested something to do, he would go along with it, even if he didn't want to do it. He would go along with it but he would complain consistently throughout the whole time when we were doing whatever it was. For example, one time we went to the beach. He didn't particularly like the beach and so he would complain that it was too hot, that there wasn't much to do and wonder when we would leave. Therefore, it caused me to not be able to enjoy my time there. I became anxious, I couldn't relax and enjoy the time that I was spending on the beach. I was trying to read a book and I could not focus on reading because I was so focused on him not being happy and wanting to leave. Therefore, it put a time restraint on my enjoying the time there. I was not able to live in the moment.

Eventually, when our relationship ended, I made myself go to all the places that I had gone to with him by myself. I was rediscovering the things that I enjoy with myself. It was hard. It was emotional because every relationship you choose to be in, there are positive moments. It's not all "bad." It's not all negative. It was a little hard emotionally but I did it. I felt so much better. I felt so much better because I discovered who I was and what made me happy. Every experience is an experience that you can take to add to who you are, to what you believe and to how you feel. I can now look at this relationship and this person with gratitude. I am thankful for this experience because I have learned a lot about myself, what I want in a relationship and what I don't want. I have sent this person and am still sending him love in the hopes that he will find himself in a beautiful relationship where he can allow himself to experience an intense intimate connection with another soul, where both of them grow together and are happy.

Forgiveness and love are essential in freeing your heart from any pain that a past relationship may have caused you. When you forgive and send love, you are connecting to your true essence, which is love, so that you may experience and draw to you the soul that you desire.

I took that experience and I made a decision with myself that I will never choose to be with somebody and remain with somebody if I am not happy. If that person is not treating me with love and respect consistently, I will not accept that relationship. Remember you cannot change someone. If you find yourself wanting to change the person you are with, you are with the wrong person. If you choose to be with someone that you wish was not a certain way, and that person is not that way, you are loving another person, not the person you are with. Therefore, why limit that person from experiencing love and why limit yourself from experiencing the love that you want? Fall in love with the person as she is.

If you love the person as she is, you won't be disappointed when she acts a certain way because you love her. You love that person as she is, not as how she could be or how you want her to be. Why love an image and not who you are with? Why love an image of what you want and not that person if it is *not* that person? Put that image out into the universe and let that soul come to you so you can love *that* soul, the soul that you love. You can't change someone. If you find yourself wanting to, you are with the wrong person. On the reverse side, if you are with someone who wants you to be a certain way, and she loves an image of someone else and not who you are, then she is with the wrong person. It is better to just let this person go so she can find the person she wants and you can have the love that you want.

It has always been the time to let go of any relationship that is not serving you. Relationships are meant to be for your highest good. If it is draining you, if it is causing a lot of resentment, a lot of pain, and you are not allowing your selves to see eye to eye, if there is no common values, you are with the wrong person. It has always been the time to let go of an abusive relationship.

♥

Do you feel that you are not good enough? All that you are is good enough. You are beautiful whether you believe it or not. You have all that you need whether you believe it or not. You are never alone whether you believe it or not. You are not your past whether you believe it or not. You do not need anyone to be happy whether you believe it or not. You are good enough. You have all that you need. When you believe that you are not good enough, you then put that energy out into the universe. You then attract people who also treat you like you are not good enough. That is not what you want to attract so therefore, you need to change that thought within yourself.

You are as beautiful as you allow yourself to feel. Other people will view you by the energy that you put out into the universe. If you believe that you are not beautiful, that's the energy that you are releasing and that people are reading from you. Those you come in contact with will sense that and consciously or unconsciously start treating you in that way. How can you be upset with someone if they treat you as you are treating yourself?

To change that, to not have people treat you in the way you do not want to be treated, you need to change that energy which you are emitting out into the universe. To do that, you need to say some affirmations with yourself.

This will allow you to begin to change the thoughts you think of every day that are inside of you. You are beautiful. You have enough. You deserve love. You do not need anyone to be happy. You are never alone. Loneliness is an illusion, it's all in your mind. You are good enough. You have all that you need. All that you desire is coming to you. You have all that you need. Just believe.

Write down the affirmative positive statements above in the first person. Ex. You are beautiful = I am beautiful.

Truths

You have all that you need.
You don't need anyone to be happy.
You are never alone.
You are good enough.
All that you desire is coming to you.
You deserve love.
You are beautiful.
You are never alone.

Affirmations

Let's talk about being comfortable in your own skin, allowing for you to be happy with yourself. When you are with yourself doing something, are you allowing yourself to truly *be* in your own company or are you indirectly with somebody else? For example, cell phones are a huge commodity in our society now: not only can you talk to somebody but you can also text somebody. When you are by yourself, when you are at the park reading, at the gym exercising, are you fully with yourself and doing that activity? Are you texting somebody or on the phone with someone? If that's the case, then you are truly *not* being with yourself. If you can do these things with your phone off or your phone not even with you, and there is no time limit that you are giving yourself because you have to go and talk to somebody, then you are at the place of just being, just *being*, with yourself.

I was at the gym the other day. I was on the treadmill, my phone was off and it was in my car. There were two people next to me, one on the left and one on the right and someone in front of me. The person on the left was talking on his phone. The person on the right was talking on his phone and the woman in front of me was texting somebody on her phone. Your exercise time is an activity that you do with yourself. Exercising is something that you allow yourself to do because you want to feel good and it is for the benefit of your health. It's an activity that you do with yourself for yourself. If you can't do that exercise for yourself and be with yourself, in just your own presence, and be ok with that, then you aren't allowing yourself to be happy in your own company. Being happy in your own company is essential for the manifestation of your Soul Mate within your life.

You need to be operating from that place of comfort with yourself. Have you found yourself hanging out with a friend, spending time with a friend and that friend is texting somebody while they are hanging out with you? Have you found yourself having a conversation on the phone with someone while you are with another friend? Our society has made it so easy to get hold of us with a cell phone at anytime of the day, night or no matter what it is we are doing. That can be a good thing in regards to an emergency. I recommend you having your cell phone, especially if you have children, in case there is an emergency. However, when you need to be talking to somebody else when you are with somebody else, you are *not* being in the moment with that person.

There is a lie in our world that we have chosen to believe. That belief is that there is not enough time. As a result, we have to bombard our moments with everything because we are not going to have enough time or we believe we are not going to have enough time. The truth is when you allow yourself to be in the moment, you relax. You remain calm. You come from a very calm, peaceful place inside of you. When you are operating from that place, there are no time restraints. You don't feel like you have to rush: you have to do this, you have to do that, you have to do this, you have to do that. You allow yourself to just *be*. When you allow yourself to just be, miraculously you feel you have plenty of time. There is no obligation. You don't have to do anything that you do not enjoy.

As a matter of fact, we tend to do a lot of things that we don't enjoy doing. We put an obligation on ourselves to do certain things because we feel that people require it of us but yet we are the only ones requiring it. We can change that requirement by recognizing how we feel. How can you recognize how you feel if you don't allow yourself to be in the moment with yourself and with whomever you are spending time with? Get rid of technology when it prohibits you from doing this.

Here's another example. Let's say you are making love with your partner. Would you be texting someone or talking on the phone while you are doing this? Why? Why would you not be doing that? Because you want to experience the pleasures of being in the moment, within *all* the moments of this experience. You want to listen to the sound of your partner's breathing, you want to feel every instance of the person's skin on yours, of being one together: every movement, every sound, every feeling. Why cheat yourself out of the pleasure of doing whatever it is you are doing as you are doing it just because you are doing it on your own, or because you place unnecessary obligations upon your time?

If you are exercising, if you are taking a walk down the street, anything that you are doing, just be and experience all the pleasures in that moment. Why take all those pleasures away by being on the phone, by distracting yourself from the present moment? When you allow yourself to be in the moment with yourself, and you don't put any time restraints on your own company or anybody else's, then you are operating from a calm place where you can be happy in the moment with yourself and with anyone you are spending time with. It's always been the time to let go. It's always been the time to let go of the need to be available at anytime for others. You have the right because you are a spiritual being, because you are a *being*. You have the right to *be*. You can truly allow yourself to be. You are the only one who can allow yourself to be. Allow yourself to bask in the excitement and the pleasure of being.

We say we waste time, but that is impossible. We waste ourselves.
~Alice Boch

Have you ever found yourself passing a couple who are expressing their love to each other? They are holding hands, embracing each other, kissing, laughing, any expression of happiness together. Have you ever passed that couple or other couples like this and felt resentment? Have you felt that those people are lucky and wondered why you can't be like that? Have you ever wondered if love will ever find you, if you will ever experience love like that? Have you ever asked yourself if you will always be unhappy? When you have those questions, when you are feeling resentment towards that couple, it is a clue that you are not happy with yourself. You are not happy with where you are in life. You are not happy with your life. The next step you need to take from there is to realize that happiness comes from within you. If you are not feeling happy, then it is something that you need to change.

Take a look at your life. Take a look at your job. Take a look at what you do outside of your job. Take a look at the people in your life. Focus on these things. How do they make you feel? When you are doing something, anything that you do outside of work or during work with yourself, just you, are you happy? It could be anything. It could be taking a walk. It could be looking at the trees blowing in the wind. It could be exercising, watching a movie, anything that you do and enjoy doing with yourself.

The truth is when you are operating from a place of calm within you and peace knowing that your Soul Mate is on his way to you, and that you do not need anything outside of yourself to be happy, you will see this couple and you will not look at them with resentment. You will be happy for their happiness. You will know that your moment of that Soul Mate love is on its way to you. That happiness with another soul is on its way to you.

Let's focus on the particular things in your life right now that may not allow you to be happy. Let's focus on the job. What do you do for a job? Is it merely a job or is it something that fulfills your inner purpose, fulfills you? Write your profession down: the title and what it is that you do.

Current Job/Career Exercise

Title   *Description*

Take a look at it. How do you feel? If it doesn't make you feel good, take a moment to write down a few things that you might like to do for a job, that you feel would be fulfilling for you. Write down as many things as you'd like.

Desirable Career/Job

Think about what you would need to go about doing these jobs. Do you have a degree in English and you would like to be a journalist or work for a newspaper? Then that's a possibility although *anything* is a possibility, even if you do not have the background for the job. If you have the passion within your heart and you want to go ahead and do this career, there will be a way for it to happen. That is how the law of attraction works. That's how the universe supports you. When you put out the intention of what you want to do, and you feel that energy behind it, that excitement, that good feeling, the universe will support you. There will be a way shown to you.

Now let's focus on the things that you do outside of work. What type of extracurricular activities do you like to do by yourself? Focus on just you. Have you ever gone to a movie by yourself? Have you ever gone out to dinner by yourself? Have you ever went to the park by yourself, opened a book and just read? Have you ever just sat down and relaxed to enjoy the energy of being outside, of being with nature, of just being? What is it that you like to do on your own? Even if you have not done any of these things that you like to do on your own but with other people, still write down the things that you enjoy doing.

Activities I like to Do

When you get to a place of being able to go and do these things on your own, and be happy and have fun, you are in the energy field of attracting your Soul Mate to you. You can do things on your own and have a wonderful time. You can do anything and have a wonderful time. Happiness comes from within you. You bring happiness to anything you experience, to anything that you do.

What about the people in your life? Let's take a look at them. Is there anybody in your life that you feel does not benefit you? In other words, the energy of that person brings you down. There is no equal give and take, a seesaw like effect where there is balance. Take a moment and think about these people. Think about everybody in your life. Write down the names of the people that you feel energized after talking to or being with. Write down on the other side the people that drain you after talking to them or being with them.

People in My Life

Positive   *Negative*

Take a look at your list. How does it make you feel? When you say the person's name, you will have a feeling behind that name. Focus on that. Now in this time of transitioning to continuously be positive and to have a positive energy field, to make these changes within yourself and your life, you are going to need to limit your time with the people that drain you. Eventually, you can still, if you choose to, have these people in your life. However, you will have to learn how to protect yourself in a way, to not let their energy seep into you and change your own. But for right now, you are going to want to limit your time with these people so that you can be around the people who are supportive of your change and who also view life as positive. It is essential to surround yourself with people who will help you elevate your energy and vice versa.

Take a look again at your list of the things that you enjoy doing. Set a little schedule for yourself. At least do one of these things per week on your own. Go out and watch a movie on your own. Go to the park, read a book on your own. Listen to music, whatever you like to do. Go shopping on your own. Go get your nails done. Go to the gym and exercise. Take yourself out to dinner. Keep a little journal. After you do these activities on your own, write down how you felt. Pay attention to how you feel. Your emotions are a very strong indicator of how you are feeling and help you to recognize the energy within you. If you are feeling good, you are operating on a very positive frequency and therefore emitting positive energy. If you are not feeling good, you are on a negative vibration. You will then attract negative energy back to you. You want to be aware of how you feel.

Loneliness is an illusion. You are never alone even when you are in your own company. When you are feeling loneliness, you are sending a negative vibration. This creates a negative energy field around you that you are putting out into the universe and therefore, attracting people that also feel lonely to help you stay in that feeling of being lonely. You don't want that. You want to get rid of loneliness. After you do these activities, write down what you feel. Focus on how you felt doing whatever it was that you were doing. When you are outside taking a walk, breathe in the air, feel the breeze on your skin. You are alive. You can allow yourself to be more alive with every moment.

♥ Time is eternal and is therefore always in the moment. Death is not an end as marriage is not an end. Love is always and will evermore be consistently existing.♥
~Gabriella Hartwell

Releasing the Past

It is always important to know when something has reached its end. Closing circles, shutting doors, finishing chapters, it doesn't matter what we call it; what matters is to leave behind us in the past those moments in life that are over.
~Paulo Coelho, <u>The Zahir</u>

♥

You have come to where you are in your life now because of all that you have experienced leading up to this moment. Your past has been an elemental part of shaping you into the person that you are, as well as who you will become. Along the way, you may have had some challenges in the form of situations and also with people. You have always had more than enough strength to get through all that you have, as well as all that you will encounter. Recognize this truth and allow yourself to be thankful for where you are in your life now as well as the person that you are.

If you hold onto the past and bring it into the present with you, your path becomes blocked. Therefore, your future will be tainted with all of the emotions you want to let go of. You will be consistently keeping company with people you no longer physically have in your life. The people that are not in your life are not in your life for a reason. What is the point of holding onto their energy?

It is ok to remember them, to be aware of the lessons you learned from your relationships, and also how you have grown as a result. This is the purpose of relationships – to learn, to grow, to allow your soul to evolve. To truly let yourself move on and have the love you deserve, you need to let go of the past: all of the people that were in your life, all of the situations that challenged you, all the tears you may have cried. Let them all go. Bless them, be thankful, and let go. It has always been the time to let go.

Forgiveness is an essential part of letting go. Therefore, can you recall a person and/or situation that comes to mind from your past that still creates pain and discomfort when you think of her or the situation?

Do you feel as though you have forgiven everyone involved? How about yourself? You can have forgiveness, even if the person you need to forgive is not in your life anymore. Perhaps your relationship ended with this person and you have both moved on or perhaps this person has abruptly left this physical world. Whatever the specific details are, you have the ability to forgive him so that the discomfort and hold on your life can be released. In addition, you can also forgive yourself, which will then allow you to truly realize and connect with the love inside yourself. You deserve to be forgiven and this person also deserves to be forgiven. We are all beings of light. There is always a purpose, a reason for every relationship we encounter. We have to distinguish what that lesson is, take it with us while at the same time letting go of any negative emotions we may have inside for what happened. It has always been the time to let go.

This forgiveness exercise is very important. Forgiving is very important: forgiving yourself and forgiving anyone that you feel has done you wrong in some way. If you do not allow yourself to forgive yourself and/or anyone else, your heart is not open. Your heart is not open to feel the love inside yourself *for* yourself. It's also not open to experience and feel the love of your Soul Mate. As I mentioned before, it's very important to be able to connect with the love inside of you, your self love for who you are in order to connect with your Soul Mate. His energy is within you. You need to connect and remember in order to draw him to you.

Forgiveness is an important part of the manifestation process. If you do not forgive, you then hold resentment towards the person that you are not forgiving and also towards yourself. There is no need to resent anything that you have done or not done. You need to forgive any activity that you have done, any words that you have said. Truly let it go. As you do this, you will see a huge result. You will feel free. You will see how you are able to notice all the beautiful things in life. You are allowing yourself and your heart to open, to feel. You block yourself from feeling when you do not forgive, when you hold resentment. Think about the person that you may still be holding some negative emotion for. It's a twofold thing because you are not allowing yourself to release that person since you are holding resentment inside. That resentment blocks your heart from being open and to truly feel, which is essential for drawing your Soul Mate to you. The other part of this is that you are, whether it be unconsciously or consciously, sending that energy to this particular individual even if they are no longer in your life. Therefore, on some level, you are prohibiting them from being completely open to experience love. When you forgive another person, you allow that person, that person's heart to open and heal. The healing is very important for the manifestation of your Soul Mate.

You can forgive someone and not forget but the forgiveness part is essential. Remember who that person truly is. We are all angels. We are all beings of light. We may not always do light filled things or say light filled words. The truth is we are all beings of light. Therefore, nothing this person said or did is personal against you. It was just a reaction. It can be released. Forgive. It has always been the time to let go of anything that is holding you back. It has always been the time to let go of anything that is holding you back from opening your heart to the love you desire.

Forgiveness Exercise

Allow yourself to envision what this person looks like. Close your eyes and imagine the smile on this person's face. Remember what it is that attracted you to him. Think of all the positive qualities that you enjoyed. Feel the emotions behind the connection you had. Slowly let your mind drift to what occurred that changed the relationship. Remember what was said and how he reacted but this time, merge all of the good qualities in. See the smile, hear the love in the voice, feel the love inside him.

Speak these words: <u>**Name of the person here**</u>**, I love you. I see the truth of who you are, which is love. I know that the words you said to me and the actions you expressed to me were not meant to hurt me. You are love. I clearly see your smile and feel the sincerity in your voice. I forgive you <u>name of the person here</u>. I release you. Be at peace.**

We are all comprised of energy. We are all connected so understand that the words you spoke and the intention behind them were sent to the person you sent them to. It is now time for you to give yourself the same beautiful and healing energy. Close your eyes, take a deep breath.

Speak these words: <u>**Your name here**</u>**, I hear the words that were spoken and I feel the pain within them. I acknowledge where I was in my life at the time I reacted in this way. I realize that this was not who I am. I forgive you for the words, the actions, the emotions that surrounded you. You are love. You deserve love. You deserve respect, most especially from me. I release this experience so that you can heal and accept the love you deserve. <u>Your name here</u>, I forgive you and let go.**

Challenges make you stronger and allow you the chance to connect with the love inside of yourself so that you can give that unconditional love to yourself. Then you will be ready to share it with someone else. There is always light within the darkness, there are lessons to be learned and parts of you that become healed. Through tears, you cleanse a part of your soul as you release the poison inside that you may have kept there for some time. Clarity and understanding can be found in your challenges. You are offered a chance to grow, and in that growth you connect to the strength within. All the challenges you have experienced in your past have shaped you into the person you are now. As you let them go, you open the doors to the future, allowing the love you desire to come to you.

♥ *To forgive is the highest, most beautiful form of love. In return, you will receive untold peace and happiness.*
~ Dr. Robert Muller ♥

Releasing the Future

You can't change the past, but you can ruin the present by worrying about the future.
~Anonymous

♥

    It is important to be in the present moment and to let go of the past but you must also let go of the future. You can have an idea where you are heading towards and I strongly recommend it, however your focus needs to be in the present. The universe is always sending you signs to guide you along your path and if you were not allowing yourself to be in the present, you may miss those signs.

    It is important to let go of the future in the way that you are not constantly focusing on it but you know where you want to go in your future. However, there is another part of this that is important. Is there any fear when you think about the future? Do you have feelings of doubt or any feelings of fear on how things will turn out, whether it be in your relationship or relationships, in your career, anything? What are you afraid of in the future? Write this down. Perhaps it is financial concerns.

Fears Regarding my Future

Take a look at your list. What about those things are you afraid of? If it's financial concerns, what about your finances are you afraid of? Now, turn these fearful things into affirmations, positive statements. If you are afraid of not having enough money to buy a house, change it around by saying, *"I will have enough money to buy my dream house."* These affirmations are going to change the energy within these fears. It's going to confirm positive energy within you. That is where you want to be when you look at these things.

Another thing is if you don't ever experience failure, or things not working out as you expected, then you will never truly be able to experience and appreciate when things do work out. There are lessons to learn in everything. Let's take a look at the word failure. Failure is a state of mind. It's what you believe about something not working out that makes it a failure or not. Failure means something that you have tried, something you may have wanted to turn out a certain way and it didn't turn out that way. Ok, what's wrong with that? Maybe it wasn't supposed to turn out that way or perhaps it was not the right time for it to turn out that way. More than likely, you have learned something from that "failure." Now you know you don't want to go about doing that particular thing the way you were attempting. Now you know what you want to try the next time. Each supposed failure makes you stronger, makes you grow and also helps you to learn. When you change the way you look at failure as the way something turns out, then there is *no* such thing as failure.

Failure is such a strong word. It makes it permanent. Something you perceive as failing, as having failed is just something that didn't work out a certain way at that time. These challenges do not mean that you have not succeeded. It means that you have grown and you have now added more to who you are. You have added more to your personality so therefore you can take that experience into the next step, the next part of your future to create what it is you want to create the way that you want to do it.

Take a look again at your list. Take each one of these things separately.

Visualization of your Future

Close your eyes, take a breath and envision your future. Envision your future step by step. Take the first thing on your list. If it is finances, look in the future to how you want things to turn out. How do you want your finances to be? Let yourself be in that moment and feel the emotions of how you want it to be like.

Think about the love that you want and the connection that you want with this Soul Mate. Envision it. Feel like you will feel *in* that moment. Take a deep breath and allow yourself to be in these visions. See the future how you want it to look like, but more importantly, focus on the feeling in those moments, how you will feel when you are living in the future you envision for yourself. It is through those intense feelings that you create what it is you want.

Releasing the Pain

Pain is Self Chosen.
~Mad Season
♥

    I mentioned how important it is to let go of your past and to let go of the future in distracting you from living in the moment, but also the fear of your future dreams not working out. These types of fears can create pain. Pain lets you know that something in your life is not working. It may be something physical. You may have a physical pain in your body somewhere. It may be creating some type of disease or some type of health problem. That pain is there for a reason. It is your job to find out what is causing you this pain.

    There may be something in your life, such as consistent thought patterns that are negative and harmful to you, that is causing your body to react in a certain way, to develop something so that it comes to your attention that there is something you need to look at. There is something that may need your attention so that you can change it. If you are exercising and you experience a very sharp pain because you were taking your body too far where it was not supposed to go yet, that pain would cause you to stop, to stop the exercise so that you can heal.

It is the same thing with any health problem that may have developed in your body for some reason. When you notice it, it is your job to sit back, notice the pain, allow yourself to feel it and then distinguish where it may be coming from. What is causing you this pain? What part of the body is it in?

A lot of our pain can be healed by our selves. We have to believe it, we have to have the strength to go beyond the pain and realize and discover what it is that is causing the pain so that we can then heal it and allow our selves to heal.

What are you holding onto that causes you pain? Is pain itself keeping you in its arms? Are you thriving on pain? Write down what it is that is causing you pain. This can be a combination of things. It can be actual physical pain that you are experiencing in your body. It can also be emotional pain. If you are not aware of what is causing you pain or where it is coming from, then write down when you experience the pain, what you are doing when you experience the pain, who you are around when the pain comes on, what you are thinking and feeling when you experience the pain.

Things That Are Causing me Pain or When I Experience Pain

Take a look at your list. Why do you think you are experiencing this pain? Maybe you had a troubled relationship and you have broken up, are feeling lonely and missing that person. Perhaps you have a lot of pain and depression, not wanting to be alone. If you stay in that state and allow yourself to feel that, and continuously feel that, and focus on those feelings, you are going to cause situations, people and circumstances in your life for you to experience more of that pain. If you attract another relationship, it is going to be with someone else who is having some type of pain or feeling lonely as well. Coming together with this person will intensify your pain. Focusing on the pain will only create more pain within your experience of life.

It is important to think about the pain in the way of trying to heal it because you have to focus on it in order to figure out where it is coming from. The unhealthy way of focusing on the pain is stating that it is always going to be there, that it is the way it is. For example, making statements like, *"I always have headaches. I am always going to have headaches,"* will keep you in the place of always experiencing headaches. But looking at the headaches to try to see what you are doing that is causing the headaches, what you are not doing that is causing the headaches, where the headaches may be coming from, why they are created in your body, then helps you to take the action so that you don't do the things that creates the headaches. It gives you motivation to make sure that those headaches don't come back so that you don't experience them anymore.

With any pain, you can let go of that relationship to it. If it is emotional pain, realize why you are still feeling it. If it is because you are afraid of being alone and you miss the feeling of companionship, make a statement with yourself that you are going to be experiencing love again. The ending of a relationship is not that you won't experience love again. It is that now you are closer to experiencing a more profound love, a more profound connection with somebody in a deeper way.

Most of the time physical pain is associated with some type of emotional pain. You may find that these are interconnected. Are you staying in a place of physical pain so that you don't have to deal with some emotional pain that you are holding inside? Perhaps there are people that have caused you some pain and instead of confronting and dealing with that pain, you keep it inside. The result of doing this is going to be some type of physical pain within your body. It is not always easy to confront the issues and/or the people that have caused you pain, however by releasing this pain, you open yourself to enjoying and experiencing all of life. Why limit yourself because of something that you have perhaps taken personally that was not meant to be taken that way? Remember what I said about people reacting from a place that they know? Well if something that they have said or done is taken from their experience or judgment of life, why take it personally within your own life? Release it and let yourself live. You are meant to be free and to allow yourself to enjoy life.

Write an affirmation or write more than one affirmation if you have some emotional pain and you also have some physical pain. Write an affirmation for all of the pain that you are experiencing to change the energy around the pain to positive energy. For example, *I will always have headaches = I will let go of this headache so that I can experience life. This headache is leaving me already. I feel it lifting away from me, releasing its hold on my body. I can breathe. My body is relaxed. I am free.*

Another example, *the companionship that I crave, that I am missing, is coming to me. As I am happy in my own presence and with myself, that love is coming to me. I can feel the love. I can feel the happiness.*

Affirmation to Release Pain

You have experienced this pain and all the pain that you have experienced for a reason. Thank the pain for being there, for giving you the chance to see that you do not want to experience it any longer. Thank the pain for allowing you to see how beautiful life is without it. Release it and let go. It has always been the time to let go.

Write a statement of gratitude for the pain. For example, if you have a pain in your heart, from a breakup, you can say, *"I am thankful for the pain I feel in my heart. It has helped me to realize my own strength. It will help me to truly appreciate the love that is coming when it is here. I am thankful. Now that I see why I had to experience this pain, I let it go. I release you and let you go."*

If there is more than one type of pain that you are experiencing, write a statement of gratitude for each one. Thank it for being there, for giving you the chance to see that you do not want to experience it any longer. Thank the pain for allowing you to see how beautiful life is without it. Thank it for giving you the experience it has given you so that you can move forward now. Release it and let go. It has always been the time to let go.

The Power of Gratitude

All that you need to love is in front of your eyes.
~Josh Groban
♥

In order to attract positive things into our lives, it is important to be in a state of gratitude. It is important to be thankful for what it is that we currently have in our lives, to be thankful for where it is that we are in our lives, who we are, all that we have experienced; the things that we may have perceived as "bad," as well as good.

When you are in a state of gratitude, you are sending out positive waves of energy into the universe. That will only bring back to you positive waves of energy. When you are being thankful for everything that you have in your life and thankful for every experience that you have had, you are allowing yourself to be happy. You are allowing yourself to be in the moment. Being in the moment will offer you more things that you can be thankful for, that you can be grateful for. You will be able to look around you and see all that you have, all that you are, all that you have experienced to make you who you are, as wonderful. Everything is as it should be NOW.

What things in life do you find beautiful? Write down what it is that you find beautiful. It could be anything: the feel of the wind on your skin, bright flowers, the smell of perfume, anything that you find beautiful, that you enjoy in life.

The Things I Find Beautiful

Take a look at your list. Do you allow yourself to appreciate these things on a day to day basis? If you don't, I would make it a priority to look at these things and notice them. Allow yourself to notice them and to appreciate them as you notice them. You will realize that there is so much that is beautiful. There is so much to appreciate that is beautiful in life. When you can appreciate the beautiful things, you realize that so many things are beautiful. Your vision on "simple" things will change. Therefore, the universe will bring more beautiful things to you.

How about the things in your life that you are thankful for? What are you thankful for in your life? It could be that you are able to wake up in the morning in a healthy state, breathing. You are able to breathe. You have a roof over your head. Whatever it is that you are thankful for in your life, write it down.

What I Am Thankful For in My Life

Take a look at your list. Do you allow yourself to be thankful for these things consistently? If you wrote down the ability to breathe, you can wake up in the morning and pay attention to your breathing. You can say, *"I am thankful that I can breathe, that I am alive."* Find ways to show the people and the things that you appreciate in your life that you are thankful for them. When you are showing that you are thankful for these things, you draw more of that energy back to you. If it is a person that you are thankful for and you are expressing that gratitude towards this person, this person will want to show gratitude for you. It is a consistent cycle of an equal balance of give and take, of appreciation.

If it is other things that you are thankful for, like the ability to breathe, then you will feel better because you will be focusing on the wonderful things of life; that you are alive, that you are breathing, that you are healthy. You will feel better when you focus on those things. That feeling better will give you inspiration to act in so many areas of your life in a positive way. You will be drawing positive people to you because of the positive energy that you will be releasing into the universe. You will then attract your Soul Mate who will also be very thankful for everything that she has in her life. She will be drawn to you because you will be thankful for all you have in your life. You will be expressing that gratitude. When you come together, you will be able to express that gratitude of life together. That will be powerful.

What challenges are you thankful for? Write a list. This could be anything like being homeless for a short period of time or perhaps you had financial difficulties. Those are challenges. It was a challenge at the time. It may have not seemed so wonderful at the time you were in that challenge. However, now when you look at it in a positive light and see the lesson you have taken from it as well as the growth you experienced, the beauty of that experience is evident. What challenges are you thankful for?

Challenges I Am Thankful For in My Life

Take a look at your list and allow yourself to feel all of the emotions that you have when you look at each one of those challenges that you are thankful for. You may have some mixed emotions. You may feel some of the same emotions you felt at the time you were experiencing the challenge however you also are feeling grateful for that. You may be feeling the positive gratitude of having that experience for it has helped make you the person that you are now. It also helps you to appreciate what you currently have in your life that much more because you can remember how it felt when you did not have those certain things or people. You then no longer take anything for granted.

Let's do an affirmation. Allow yourself to say these words below:

I am thankful for the challenges I have experienced in my life. These challenges have brought me to where I am right now in my life. These challenges have made me who I am right now in my life. I am thankful for these challenges. They are a part of me, and for that, I am thankful.

I want to relay an experience I had which is a beautiful example of being thankful and expressing gratitude in the midst of experiencing a challenge. I was at Starbucks with my laptop writing this book. There was a homeless woman outside. This was a very hot day. She was outside sitting at a table eating beans from a can. Someone had given her some money so she had come in to get a frappacino of some sort. She came in and right when she came in, she closed her eyes and she put her arms out. She said, *"This is heaven."* She was thankful for the cool air in Starbucks.

After she got her drink, she went back outside, continued eating her beans. She would then take a break from eating her beans, and she would start dancing. Starbucks was playing music which could be heard from outside. She was dancing and she was a very good dancer. She was having such a good time. She was truly being in that moment, dancing.

She would then take a break from dancing and she would get on her knees. She would lift her hands and her arms up to the heavens. She would look up to the sky and she said, *"Thank You."* She took her hand, kissed it and then extended it to the heavens again. She clasped her hands in a prayer position and closed her eyes. She then stood up, sat down and continued eating.

She kept doing this. She would take a break from eating, start dancing again and she would express her gratitude again. Also, she would hold the door open for people coming into or out of Starbucks. There were other people that went outside to sit outside and she would offer her chair. She gave somebody her chair and went to get another chair for herself. She would watch people as they expressed love to each other and she smiled. She had a huge smile on her face when she was watching others give love. There were times when she was dancing and people would approach her and smile or say something and she would laugh.

Focus on the experience that I have just shared with you as an example of gratitude. What was this homeless woman being thankful for?

<u>The Things This Homeless Woman was Thankful For</u>

Take a look at your list. Are any of those things that she was thankful for you are also thankful for? Have you ever allowed yourself to feel thankful for those things? Have you allowed yourself to be thankful for being alive, being able to breathe and to walk and to dance? Have you allowed yourself to feel thankful for having food and a drink, a *cool* drink on a *hot* day? Have you allowed yourself to be thankful for having clothes on your back, having air conditioning on a very hot day or being able to walk into a place that has air conditioning to cool off for a while? Have you allowed yourself to be thankful for the expression of love even if it is not being displayed directly to you? Have you allowed yourself to feel thankful for the ability to give?

Giving and being kind to others is a powerful action because it only goes back to you, the giver. You receive so much by giving to somebody else. You feel the power of your own love and your own worth. Gratitude is a very powerful thing.

I also want to mention how people reacted to this homeless woman as she was dancing and as she was being grateful. Most people express their gratitude in a place where they are away from other people so others are not witnessing their expression of gratitude, of being thankful. This woman was doing it out in the open where anybody could see her.

As she was dancing, people looked at her as if there was something strange about her. Yet those same people that looked at her strange, changed the way they reacted to her when she was kind to them, when she opened the door for them and offered her chair. They then looked at her as if she was just expressing herself. Their attitude changed.

There is nothing unusual or strange about enjoying life and being in the moment, no matter what it is you are doing. If you aren't disrupting somebody else from being able to do that as well, then there is nothing wrong and nothing unusual about that expression.

Imagine how it would be if we consistently looked at those types of things with love rather than fear or restriction? We would be living in heaven so to speak, heaven on earth. Why is it that those people changed their attitude after she was kind to them? Why did they look at her differently?

<u>Why the Difference in Attitude?</u>

There are lots of judgments that we make unconsciously. When we experience anything, when we observe people, when we observe situations, when we observe ourselves, we are making opinions about ourselves and about others. As I mentioned there are only two emotions: fear and love. Our opinions either come from either fear or love. The opinions that come from fear are because of something we have unconsciously decided to believe. In relation to the above example, it could be a general assumption we have chosen to adopt about homeless people. Homeless people are not alcoholics. Homeless people are not particularly homeless because they want to be. There have been circumstances that have happened to them that have caused them to be that way. Can they get out of that situation? Yes they can. When they are ready and they choose to, they can get out of that situation. However, they also grow through that situation. As you can see, the situation for this woman has allowed her to appreciate the very simple things in life, like living in the moment, appreciating all the little things in life: being able to eat, being able to breathe, being able to drink, being able to feel the air on her skin. If she was not in her situation, she may not have experienced those things like she has.

When we don't judge people and experiences that we have and we let go of fear, it is a whole different experience. How much we can learn and gain from the experience of watching this woman when we are not afraid of her or what she may represent in our world? If there are kids watching this woman, that is wonderful. Why instill in our children fear that we may have taken on as we grew up? They should be able to feel that if there is a song that comes on and they are outside, they can dance to it. They can enjoy that song, to feel the beat, feel the rhythm, feel the energy of that song and not worry about what someone else will think. There is nothing wrong with expressing yourself. It is fear that stops us from enjoying all of those things.

Are there any other things that you would like to write down now that you are thankful for that you may have forgotten? Write another list now of all the things that you are thankful for.

Things That I Am Thankful For

Allow yourself to feel all the emotions when you think about all these things. How is gratitude important in drawing your Soul Mate to you? This homeless woman who was feeling and expressing her gratitude can only bring wonderful things into her life because the more people released their opinions when they looked at her, the more people wanted to talk to her. She ended up laughing and then they ended up laughing. Why? She was emitting positive energy. She was thankful for life and therefore, she brought people to her that wanted to experience the gratitude of life as well with her.

When you are being thankful for what you have in your life, and you are expressing that gratitude, you are in that positive energy field. You are then going to attract souls to you that feel the same way. Your Soul Mate will be drawn to you. Gratitude is a very essential part of drawing your Soul Mate to you. Gratitude also allows you to be happy in the moment, to be happy with yourself. Happiness draws more happiness unto itself. You will draw more people unto you that are happy as well. Your Soul Mate will be one of those people.

♥♥♥♥

Part Three: Steps to Take to Attract Your Soul Mate into Your Life

♥

♥♥♥♥

1. Believe It, Feel It, Know It, Act on It

The law of attraction states that what you put out into the universe, what you think about, what you feel about, what you act on is going to come to you. How does this relate to coming in contact with your Soul Mate? You need to know, you need to believe that this particular person you want to attract is coming to you and is on his way to you. You need to believe this without any doubt. If you believe that, if you feel that, if you are acting in that way, then there is no way that this person cannot come to you. However, instead of focusing on how you are going to get there, focus your energy more on what you are doing in your life.

Start being the person that you have always wanted to be. Do the things you have always wanted to do. Don't focus on the next step, how it's going to happen. You don't need to know these things. All you need to focus on is to know the end result: that the person you want IS coming to you. The end result is you WILL be with this person.

It's important for you to truly believe that your Soul Mate is on his way to you. In order to do this, you need to act in the way that you believe he is coming to you. You need to truly believe without any doubt that he is coming to you, that he is on his way to you *right now*. You need to feel, allow yourself to feel this.

I want to go into some detail with each of these areas because I want you to understand what this means. Let's first take acting in the way that you know he is on his way to you. Everything in your life needs to express your belief and your knowing that he is on his way to you. For example, if you have a bed that is not big enough to have someone sleeping beside you, you are not allowing that energy to be next to you. If you were to have a bed that is big enough for your Soul Mate to sleep next to you, you are opening that energy field of connection.

If your closet does not have enough space for her clothes, it is not expressing the open area to allow her to move in with you. Your environment, your surroundings need to coincide with the belief that your Soul Mate is on her way to you. You may need to make room in the place that you are currently living so that it sends a message to the universe that you are taking the steps in believing and knowing that this soul is on the way to you.

Let's talk about feeling because feeling is very attached to your surroundings as well. Feeling that he is on his way to you, and acting in that way coincide. When you feel and allow yourself to feel that he is already on his way to you, meaning that he is with you *now*, you can then feel his essence with you. This would then cause you to take the action to make room for him in your bed because you feel as if he is already there. You would then feel the desire to create space in your closet, in your apartment, in your life for him.

When you allow yourself to feel these emotions, your feelings become so strong that in a way it feels as if she doesn't even need to come because it feels as if she is already there with you. When you can feel that and you can envision her there with you that strongly, you are putting a very strong intention out into the universe. You are sending a strong message to the universe, which will only deliver this soul to you.

I want to talk about believing a little more because this is an important step in manifesting anything within your life. If you do not believe it, and you only allow yourself merely to think about it, you do not have the strength to create anything in your life. You may have heard some people say that they believe that anything is possible, except *this* particular thing. Well, let me tell you something. If you believe that anything is possible, you cannot put restrictions on that belief. It is either you believe *anything* is possible or you do not. If anything is possible, there are *no* restrictions, there are *no* limitations.

If you believe that your Soul Mate is on his way to you, you have to truly believe that. You cannot say, "*I believe that he is on his way to me, but if it doesn't happen by THIS time, then he is not coming to me.*" That is placing a restriction on your belief. You cannot believe something if you put any type of limitation on that belief. You have to trust and you have to feel, you have to act and you have to know that he is on his way to you. No matter what you experience in the time before he gets there, you have to allow yourself every day to *feel* it, to *believe* it, to *act* in that way, and to *know* it. When you have all of these emotions and actions coinciding, he will be here. You will experience that love that you are craving.

♥♥♥♥

2. Live in the Moment

It's very important that you be aware. In order to be aware, you need to be living in the moment. You can't focus on the past. You can't focus on the future. Definitely, you need to know where you are going in the future and what your intentions are. You need to know who it is you want to attract, what type of person you are attracted to, but you can't continue to focus on that. If you continue to think about this person and how you will be with her, when you will be with her, you are not living in the present. You truly need to be aware of everything that comes to you: every person that comes to you, every situation that comes to you, every thought, every feeling that comes to you.

The in between stuff will be shown to you along the way, as you are moving through your days. The middle of the road can be distracting. It can take you away from life, from living. The important thing in life is the journey, not the destination. You begin again, in a way, when you reach that destination, but life is the journey. It is very important to be in the moment. If you're not aware in the moment, you won't recognize the signs that come to you to guide you on what step to take to bring you to that person.

What does it mean to live in the moment? Well, it simply means to let go of the future and let go of the past. By letting go of the future, you are not focusing on it. You are not constantly thinking about it. You do need to know and I would recommend knowing where you feel you want to go in your future, with everything: your career, your Soul Mate (the type of person you want to attract), the type of people that you want in your life. When you are constantly thinking about your future, thinking about your Soul Mate, when you are going to meet, who it is going to be, if you are ever going to meet, it stops you from living in the present moment. It does not allow you to be happy and calm right now in the present moment. Living in the present moment is essential for the manifestation of your Soul Mate within your life. It is in the present moment that there are signs for you to follow to be guided to this person.

You can take a look at what you have in your life. You can take a look at the people you have in your life. You can take a look at yourself, your health, everything that you do have and you can choose to be happy, right now in this present moment. When you choose to be happy right now, you will see everything around you in a different light. You will be open and you will allow yourself to notice the signs that are guiding you to your Soul Mate.

What does living in the moment mean to you? Are there examples you think of? It could be walking down the street noticing the trees blowing, focusing on only the breeze on your skin. Whatever you have done or whatever comes to your mind when you think of living in the moment right now – write those things down.

Living in the Moment Exercise

      Then allow yourself to intentionally do these things. Take them one at a time. How do you feel? If it makes you feel good, you want to do these things. Deep down inside of us, in addition to our desire to be happy, we also want to just be, not having any responsibilities. This is what vacation is for. We try not to have any particular responsibilities. Sometimes we travel and we go places and in a way there is some type of responsibility that goes along with that, but for the most part, we want to get to wherever we are going on vacation and relax. We want to just be and when you are just being, you are *being* in the moment. You are allowing yourself to be in the moment. As you know, that is very important for the attraction of anything you want in your life, especially your Soul Mate.

      In addition, you need to let go. You need to let go of the result. You may have an idea of the person that is coming to you but you also have to be open to the prospect that maybe exactly what you feel is not exactly what will show up in the *way* you feel he will show up. Be aware. Be open to your answer being given in unexpected ways and unexpected places.

♥♥♥♥

3. Notice the Signs and Follow Them

How do you notice the signs? You have to get to that place of allowing yourself to be happy in the present moment, of allowing yourself to be happy now, of realizing that happiness comes from within you. You can be happy at any moment of your life. You can consistently be happy whether you are single, whether you have a perfect job at this moment, doesn't matter. What matters is that you *choose* to be happy. When you are in that moment, you are open to noticing signs. Signs are around you all the time.

There may be a particular number sequence that you see often on license plates. The angels and the universe are always speaking to us. Numbers are used to communicate messages to us. I would recommend taking a look at Doreen Virtue's *Angel Numbers* book. If there is a specific number sequence that you usually see, there is a message there. If you hear a song on the radio and when you hear the song, there is a message there. The lyrics may be the words you need to hear. When you read something, whether it be a magazine or a book, there may be a line or more than one line that speak to you. There may be someone that comes to you and says something or you overhear a conversation. There are many ways that signs come to you. When you are aware and you are living in the moment, you are able to notice those signs. Therefore, you are able to act on them.

Someone may come up to you and invite you to a party. You may meet your Soul Mate at this party. You may have wanted a particular job and then someone comes up to you or you see an advertisement of a vacancy for that specific job. It just happens to be where you are walking. Let's say you have to take a detour because there was some construction going on and then you came across this vacancy sign which you would not have come across if there wasn't construction going on. It is one thing that happens, another thing that happens and another thing that happens. It is a sequence of synchronistic things that happen so that you can get a sign. Once you notice that sign, your job is to follow it.

The universe loves you. You are part of the universe. The universe wants you to be happy. It wants to support you. If you are happy, it wants you to stay there. If you are not happy, it wants you to stay there because it's only going to react to how you are feeling, how you are *allowing* yourself to feel. If you are allowing yourself not to feel good, and you consistently stay in that place of not feeling good, then the universe is going to give you more of that because it cannot distinguish whether you want that or not. If you put your focus and your energy on it, then that is what you are putting out to the universe. Deep down inside, you know that you don't want that. You want to be happy. Deep down inside, we all want to be happy. Therefore, that is our mission. Our mission is to

BE happy. Once you accomplish being happy no matter what is going on in your life, no matter who is within your life, especially if you are single, that is the frequency that will attract your Soul Mate to you. This is also the frequency that will attract the signs to you so that you can notice and follow them to come in contact with your Soul Mate.

The Moment of NOW

I call you, dream master
I welcome you, dearest angels
to meet me in the night, when my breathing has become true
to run with me through the visions of all that is,
where the past and future merge with the present, in the NOW
teach me to rhyme as I knew when I was a child
show me how to laugh in the most profound form
connect me to the essence of all that is pure and good
it is the truth that I can be sure is within me
the presence of the divinity in the manifestation of my self.
I bow to you, dream master
I kneel at your feet, dearest angels
as your whispers greet my eager ears,
anticipating the next sign to guide me on this chosen path
be with me as my emotions calm these nerves
sit with me as I explore the nuances of the woman that is me
remind me of the beauty that breathes so naturally within me
that weaves its magic so eloquently around me
that intimately moves its presence upon me
that softly flows so deeply through me.
I thank you, dream master
I honor you, dearest angels
Experience is a strong teacher
I will heed your words, notice the signs,
follow the steps, and embrace the NOW.
The moment of now is where manifestations are born.

Part Four: What a Soul Mate Relationship Will Feel Like

Communication through respect and love is the whole key to keeping the love alive and never getting bored in your relationship.
~Don Miguel Ruiz, <u>The Mastery of Love</u>

1. Communication With Understanding and Love

When you communicate with each other, it will be out of love and respect. You will not say words that will hurt each other. You will not call each other any names that could hurt the other. Before you say something, you will *feel* it. You will then decide to change what you are going to say because of the realization that it could hurt your partner. You will be sympathetic to your partner's feelings. You want to remain in the place of love. You are always operating from a place of love with this soul. When you communicate, there will be no yelling. There will be no arguing. There will be discussions and you will both allow your selves to listen to each other, really listen to each other.

If there is something that comes up that may cause a disagreement, if you are feeling one way and your partner is feeling another way, you will allow your selves to see the other point of view, even if it is something that you don't agree with. You will respect and love your Soul Mate through this disagreement and discussion. When you do that, you will realize that the disagreement wasn't really that big of a deal. It is what you have created. Disagreements, arguments are what you create because you do not allow yourself to listen and see where the other person is coming from. When you do that, the only emotion that remains, the only energy that remains, is love.

If something is bothering you that perhaps your Soul Mate may have said or done and it has caused you to feel a certain way, instead of keeping this inside to cause resentment, you will talk to your Soul Mate about it. You will never go to bed angry. You will never allow yourself to feel consistently any type of disruption within the relationship. If there is anything that causes such a feeling, it will be discussed right in the beginning so that it can be released. The way that you communicate with this soul will be so much more evolved than any other relationship that you have had in the past. However, every relationship you have had in the past has prepared you, has made you ready for *this* relationship. Know that truth, feel that truth, be thankful for that truth.

♥♥♥♥

2. There Will Be No Doubt

When you are in the presence of your Soul Mate, there will be no doubt. You may have had relationships in the past where something was nagging at you. Some feeling was telling you this is not the person. When you got that feeling and heard those words, maybe you didn't listen. Perhaps you told yourself that you didn't know why you were feeling that way and doubted the feeling. You continued the relationship. Eventually you did realize that this person was not for you. When you come in contact with your Soul Mate, there will be no doubt. From the moment that you meet, from the moment that your energies connect, you will know. There will be absolutely no question and no doubting feelings. There will only be knowing, an *absolute* knowing.

♥♥♥♥

3. Height Will Not Be a Factor

There may have been times in the past as well as times now where you have set specific limits on the person you want to attract. Perhaps you have liked brown hair, a certain height, any particular thing you believed you wanted in the form of a material or a physical thing. Those things will not be a factor when you meet your Soul Mate. If you don't like hair on a man's chest, when you come in contact with your Soul Mate, the hair on his chest will not matter. It will transform into the most beautiful masculine trait to you. If you believe you are attracted to women with blonde hair, and your Soul Mate has brown hair, brown hair will be more beautiful to you than any other hair color. It is the person that makes those traits attractive, not the other way around. That is the truth.

In addition, if you are literally taller than your Soul Mate or he is taller than you, and you are standing in front of each other, that height will not make a difference. You will feel as if you are the same height because you are on the same level. It will feel as though nobody else is physically around you other than the two of you. Everything will disappear. Everyone around you will disappear and you will both be *completely* connected.

♥♥♥♥

Love is not to be found in someone else, but in ourselves; we simply awaken it. But in order to do that, we need the other person.
~Paulo Coelho, <u>Eleven Minutes</u>

4. You Will Be the Mirror of Each Other

When you come in contact with this Soul Mate, you will see yourself within his eyes. He will be the mirror of you, who you are. Therefore, you will begin to love yourself more as well as loving him more. It's a continuous cycle. The more that you see him being who he is, you will love who you are and in turn, love him more. He will feel the same about you. The type of need here is based on a healthy need; by being in the presence of the other person we are able to see more clearly who we are as well as the love within us. It is in the presence of this other that we have become awakened to the love and beauty within us because we see it coming from this person. As we see this, we connect with the love inside ourselves and realize that we are just as beautiful. We don't need that person to survive but with their existence and presence in our lives, we can see more clearly through the eyes of love.

There will be no doubt when you come in contact with your Soul Mate. There will be a mirror of love back to you within her eyes. You will see yourself there. You will love yourself more and you will love this soul. You will not argue. Height will not be a factor.

You will experience heaven on earth. You will feel as if every moment of your life is blissful. You may feel that you were meant to be here. You are meant to be with this person. You will connect with your true essence, which is love. You will continuously *give* love. You will always *see* love within others, within the world, within yourself. You will always smile. You will always be happy. Happy will be a consistent state.

Creativity will be consistent. You will be so inspired in so many areas of your life that you will be amazed. It will be as if you were never inspired before. You will not be able to see how you ever lived before. In a way, you won't even be able to imagine it. It may be an awakening of sorts, as a birth into this new person, into this new life, into this heaven on earth. It is what deep inside we are all striving for. We all want to feel that heaven, that heaven that we came from, that heaven that we truly never left. You will experience heaven on earth, heaven inside yourself, heaven in this person, heaven around you. You will experience heaven, heaven on earth.

♥♥♥♥

5. *There Will Be Unconditional Love*

There will be unconditional love between you and your Soul Mate. You will place no conditions on this love that you receive from this soul. You will not place any conditions on your love that you give. This person will not have to do a certain thing, say a certain thing in order for you to love him. He will not need you to do or say anything. All you need to do is be yourself. You both allow each other to be your selves with each other. There is so much freedom in that. There is so much love in allowing another person just to be who she is.

There will be *no* jealousy. Jealousy can be created for lots of reasons. You can *feel* jealousy for lots of reasons. We may choose to believe that when we get married or when we are in a committed relationship, we cannot have friends that are of the opposite sex nor can we meet new friends who are of the opposite sex. Perhaps this belief stems from the fear that there may be romantic emotions that come up as a result of this relationship. The truth is that we are all connected and we can all learn from each other. We need each other to grow. Every relationship that we have is an opportunity for us to grow. If we limit ourselves with connecting to others, we hinder our own growth.

When you connect to and are with your Soul Mate, there will be no restrictions placed on you regarding any relationship that you have or that you may have. You will be able to have friends of the opposite sex. It will actually be encouraged. Within us, we have equal parts, masculine and feminine parts. Everybody has these two sides within the psyche and it is essential to have balance. You will not have this balance if you limit yourself from having any male friends or female friends. You may have had an experience in a past relationship where the person you chose to be with was not okay with you having friends that were of the opposite sex. You just need to let that go. It has always been the time to let go of any belief that has been restricting you from truly experiencing love.

What may be causing the feeling of jealousy? Perhaps there is a belief that you are not good enough and so therefore you feel threatened by another woman or man. The truth is not that you are threatened by another woman or man, but that you feel you are not good enough, that you are not attractive enough. Why restrict the person that you love from growing in a relationship with a friend because of this belief that you have? The best thing to do would be to work with that belief within yourself and let it go. The truth is that you are good enough. You are attractive. You are a being of light. You deserve to experience love.

Another belief which connects to the previous one is the fear that this person will leave you for somebody else. This could happen. If this were to happen, then it would be what would need to happen so that you can experience the love with someone that you desire. Everything happens for a reason. Like I mentioned earlier, if you are looking for someone other than who you are with, or if the person you are with is looking for someone other than you, it's better to end the relationship. It is better to attract the person you want instead of being together and being unhappy. If that person is going to go to another woman or man, then it is going to happen. Why try to make it not happen by restricting the person's relationships?

Think of the story of Peter Peter Pumpkin Eater who had a wife and couldn't keep her. He placed her in the pumpkin so she couldn't go out or do anything. Did that serve their relationship? How do you think their relationship was? Probably it was very restrictive and suffocating, not a *relation ship* at all. When you are in your Soul Mate relationship, there will be trust. You will be able to trust that your partner can go out with his female friends for you know that he is coming home to you. You know that he loves you. There will no concern about jealousy. You will not even be jealous because deep within your soul, you know that you love each other and that your love will sustain you.

All of the friends that you have and all of the friends that you will have are a part of what make you who you are. If you restrict yourself, or if you restrict your partner from experiencing and having these relationships, you are stopping them from connecting with who they are. Connecting with who you are is so essential in a relationship because if you cannot connect with who *you* are, you will not be able to connect with somebody else that you choose to have a relationship with. Pay attention to your feelings. When you realize that you have no jealousy, you are in the presence of your Soul Mate. You know that you are truly happy with yourself, that you have a strong bond with the soul you choose to be with and there is no need at all to be jealous.

♥♥♥♥

What this marriage is intended to do, this new form of marriage, is to fuel the engine of your experience – the experience of who you really are and who you chose to be.
~Neale Donald Walsch on Relationships: Applications for Living

6. Marriage: A New Beginning

Perhaps, you have heard somebody say, *"I am not going to get married."* You may have heard somebody say, *"marriage is not any fun."* You may have heard somebody say, *"marriage places too many conditions upon who I am."* Who wants to live in a relationship with restrictions, especially forever? How do you view marriage? We have talked about this earlier. Has your view of marriage changed? Do you find it a positive commitment or a negative one? Do you feel that after a certain amount of years you will not be happy with each other anymore? Do you feel that you will be stuck in a routine that is boring and that there will be no excitement together?

Marriage was created so that we could experience the joy of *living* together, the joy of physically living together but also just being alive, *living* together. Marriage is a commitment that two souls make so that their missions are joined together. They can love each other as well as others. They can experience the joy of life, *every single thing* together.

How do you feel our world views marriage? If you have heard many people say things that are not positive in reference to marriage, why do you think that is? What are the views on marriage in our world? How we act, our traditions show us what we believe. Let's look at the bachelor and the bachelorette party. Many people choose to have these parties before getting married. What do these parties symbolize? These parties symbolize the end of freedom. It will be your last night with the girls or the last night with the guys. There is a belief that you are limiting yourself, limiting your experience of life, your experiences in general when you get married to somebody. This is the truth if you *allow* it to be the truth.

If you operate from a place of jealousy, of restrictions, of placing conditions upon each other, then it *will* be the end to your freedom. Love is not meant to be like that. Love is free. Love is open to experiencing life, all aspects of life. When you have restrictions in a relationship and conditions, how can you view that as something fun and something to commit to? If you look at it like that, you can understand why people would say that they are not going to get married. It's natural for us not to want to do something that is not fun.

Think of two people that decide to get married. They truly love each other. They allow themselves to be who they are. They allow themselves to have friends of the same and opposite sex. They allow the other to go out with their friends, away from each other, but also sometimes they go out with their friends together. They then come back to each other and share their experiences. They have grown. Through every experience, we have an opportunity to grow. We have an opportunity to add more to who we are. We can then share it with the soul that we choose to spend the rest of our lives with. In that sharing, bonds are created. Our relationship evolves. Our relationship strengthens. If we deny ourselves that, how can our relationship strengthen? It only weakens.

If you want to experience Soul Mate love for the rest of your life, if you truly desire to experience this love, change your thoughts on marriage. Marriage is not an ending. It is a beginning. Marriage is not the end to freedom. It is the beginning of a new freedom. It is the beginning of the end to conditions. It is the beginning of loving each other for who you are and who you will become.

Peace in Love

Your image emerges within my memory
I am transported to your side,
inspired by the simplicity of who I am.
The energy of you sustains me
and eases my mind into spirit.
My true nature is peace,
peace with life,
peace in love,
peace in being.
I am addicted, so to speak
as my ego becomes weak,
losing the game of tug of war.
There is strength within my being that I connect with when I look
into your eyes,
which overflow with the intensity of emotion that I feel for you
I feel of you
I feel with you
I feel beside you
I feel around you
I feel you.
You are the sanctuary I have always known,
the sanctuary I created before and after my birth.
You may say that beholding your form
and remembering the essence that is you
has been a re-birth of me.
I am transformed
I am free
I am me and you
I am me in you.

Part Five: What a Soul Mate Relationship Will Look Like

♥♥♥♥

1. Energies Will Be Similar

When Soul Mates come together, there will be some similar physical features. They may have a similar light in their eyes, their facial structure may be the same. What you will notice in a Soul Mate relationship is that the energies of both of these souls are similar. They match. They have similar values, where they want to go in life will be the same. How they treat others complements one another. The energy that they put out into the universe will be operating on the same frequency.

♥♥♥♥

2. The Presence of Love Will Be Inviting to Others

People will be drawn to them. People will want to talk to them. People will want to help them. People will just randomly say hi to them. They will want to be close to them in some form. It is very inviting to be in the presence of love. When there is love so deep that there are no judgments, the natural feeling is to want to be in the presence of that. It then allows whoever is around that type of love to feel comfortable with who they are. This type of love is so transformative for the people that are in the relationship as well as anybody else who comes in contact with them or who witnesses their relationship and their strong love. You will see these people laughing and smiling all the time. They will be expressing their love to others all the time. They will be happy just being and they will not be afraid to express who they are in any way. Because of that, others will feel comfortable to be who they are around them. This is how all the leaders who lived in love, such as Jesus and Gandhi, attracted people to follow them. It was the love within them that came out in their voice, in what they said, in the light in their eyes, how they treated others.

Love is constantly being released from two people who are in a Soul Mate relationship. Love is being released from each one individually but also together. When you see both of these souls illuminating this type of love, it is overwhelming. Some people may cry. Some people may laugh. Some people won't be able to believe it in a way because it will seem so beautiful, so good to be true.

This is another belief in our world that is not true. The belief is that something or someone can be *too good to be true*. Nothing is too good to be true, unless we believe it is. Believing that something or someone is too good to be true is because there is another belief behind it, that we don't deserve the good, the good does not last. However, if you believe in good, good can last *forever* and *never* end. If you focus on the good, the good will last and the good will never end. When you are looking at this Soul Mate couple as they are expressing and are *in* love, you realize that nothing is too good to be true. Goodness can last if you allow it. If you believe it, and if you allow it, goodness is right around the corner. Allow yourself to embrace it.

You Choose Your Destiny

♥♥♥♥

Destiny is not a matter of chance. It is a matter of choice: It is not a thing to be waited for, it is a thing to be achieved.
~ William Jennings Bryan

Destiny almost goes hand in hand when Soul Mates are discussed. When destiny is referred to, people are talking about something in life that is going to happen to you regardless of anything that you do, say, believe, think or feel. I am here to tell you that this is not the case. Is destiny part of finding your Soul Mate and being with this soul? Yes, it most definitely is.

This is the truth about destiny. You have free will. You were given free will so that you can make choices in your life. You can experience what it is that you want in life. You have the choice to create whatever destiny you wish to create. If you want to experience Soul Mate love, then you need to allow yourself to be in the moment so that you can notice the signs the universe sends to you for you to experience that love. Those signs then guide you to that person, to the destiny of being with that particular person that you want to be with.

You have a choice to take the steps once you notice the signs or not. You have a choice not to notice the signs, to block yourself from noticing them and from following them. In that case, you will not have that destiny. There are various destinies that you can experience in your lifetime, just like there are various Soul Mates that you can be with throughout your lifetime. If you want to experience the highest divine Soul Mate love, you *can* experience that love. You merely have to notice the signs and take the steps towards that destiny that you are choosing. Destiny is not something that just happens to you. You have a choice in the formation of any destiny that you experience.

You find your destiny on the road you've taken to being who you are.
~Gabriella Hartwell

Who You Are Reveals Who I Am

The light in your eyes makes me comfortable being who I am
And I am free, though the truth is that I have always been free
now I am realizing that my freedom has existed, persistent within me, all along
Touching skin is so powerful, energy exchanges that move our souls to create
And appreciate who we are, where we are, the knowledge that we are always connected,
Always connecting.
I can feel you as you are living your heart's desire – my love for you grows stronger with each breath you exhale
with each expression you reveal - I watch you from a distance
I know you with each vibration of your voice,
remembering our promise before we knew of each other in our perceived reality
reality is our souls merged together
each day that truth refreshes me – let it restore your energy too my love
I await your presence into my life.

Prayers

Prayer on Believing

I allow myself to believe
I can have anything I choose
If I believe, anything is possible
If I feel and I know, anything is possible
Anything is possible if I believe
I open myself to receive all the beautiful parts of life
Everything in life is beautiful
I allow myself to believe
I believe in the power of my dreams
I believe that I am beautiful
I allow myself the strength to believe that my Soul Mate is on the way to me
I believe I connect with the truth inside myself
and I know that love exists
Love sustains
Love is if I believe
I do
I do believe.

Prayer on Hearing your Inner Guidance/Voice

I allow myself to recognize and hear the voice within me that is guiding me
through every step I should take in life
I allow my mind to quiet so that I can hear the inner truth coming from within me
the inner truth that is guiding me
I allow myself to let go of all the distractions in my life
I will release my thoughts
I will let go of anything in material form that is in the way of my hearing
I allow myself to listen,
I allow myself to hear my inner guidance
I allow myself to connect with my inner truth.

Prayer on Being in the Moment

I allow myself to be in the moment
I allow myself to be in every single moment as I am living it
I allow myself to be in the moment without any distractions
and without any restrictions
I allow myself to be in the moment without any doubts
I allow myself to connect with the happiness within me
I create my own happiness
and I can release it to the world
I allow myself to experience every part of my day
I feel the wind on my skin
I watch the clouds move in the sky
I listen to the birds as they sing their song
I enjoy the warmth of the sun on my body
I feel my hair as it moves with the wind
I am existing right now in the moment as it is happening *right now*.

Prayer on Being Happy with Myself

I enjoy my own company
I am beautiful
I am full of love
I am love itself
I allow myself to experience anything I wish in life
If I want to go and experience something, I will do it
I do not need someone else with me to do it
I can have fun on my own
I am fun to be with
Who I am is so unique
I have so much beauty
My light shines and the world can see it
I can feel it
I allow myself to be content in my own company
I give myself love
I am love
I am ready to receive love
I treat myself as I treat others
I treat myself with love
I treat myself with respect
I love myself
I love who I am
I am beautiful
I allow myself to be comfortable in my own skin
I am who I am because I am *alive*.

Tonight, that I Might See...

My prayers have been answered
Tonight that I might see…
a vision of you before me
smiling, full of spirit
For you are the pioneer my love
The essence of you inspires
the divine within others
calls to the spirit of one
Infinity within

We are close to the sun
growing brighter each day
as one touches another
We find there is light within us all
Beauty exists as beauty persists
Beauty is real as reality is beautiful
Look to the heavens my love
The sunsets are on fire
Passion ignites us and unites us
We co-exist with nature
as nature dwells within us
We are consistently creating ecstasy between us
A new dawn emerges
breaks and re-defines who we are
because we are always changing

God says yes!
We have heard
We have remembered
It is now time to take action
and live our destiny
We can only be who we are

Hey you, yes you!
Believe in the power of your desires
They are the truths inherently breathing within you
The other side of you
awaits you
To embrace you
To accept you
To merge with you
and all you have to do is
be you
feel you

Love makes the world awake
Love makes the world true
Truth is what we seek
We are only prisoners of pain if we choose to be imprisoned
to break free only requires our time,
our focus,
our shift of consciousness

Recognize and hold onto the kiss of life
It is love
Love defined through emotion,
Experience, kindness
Love expressed through forgiveness,
Acceptance, creativity
Love exhaled through a kiss,
a touch, a smile

Tonight, that I might see…
Love is our truth
We are love
We are here to love,
to give love,
make love,
feel love,
breathe love,
be love.

Tonight, that I might see…

About the Author

Gabriella Hartwell is an Intuitive Relationship Life Coach who also receives messages from the angels and offers guidance readings. She works with individuals and couples to help them to realize and connect to the essence of love within them.

Her belief is that when the connection of love has been established, it will seep into all areas of life. Everything that once seemed dark will become illuminated. Relationships will be healed and true Soul Mate love can be known and embraced.

She is currently working on many projects to continue to bring love and light to the world. If you want her to have a book signing or a seminar near you, you may visit her website. All are welcome.

www.emergingsoul.com
Embrace your Destiny!

If you could make unlimited wishes within your experience of life, imagine how much you would be able to enjoy being *alive*? The truth is that there are no limits on your experiences except those that you place on yourself.

Go forth and allow yourself the chance to live your dreams. Allow yourself the chance to embrace the love within you, for it is the love you will attract to you.

May all the love in your heart warm you,
♥ Gabriella Hartwell ♥

Made in the USA
Lexington, KY
07 February 2011